用 多 家 朱

Chu Gar Skills

Hakka Southern Mantis Kungfu

Huizhou Chu Gar

About Wooden Man

Yellow Ox Staff

About Dui Jong

Yang Style Chu Gar

History and Pictorial

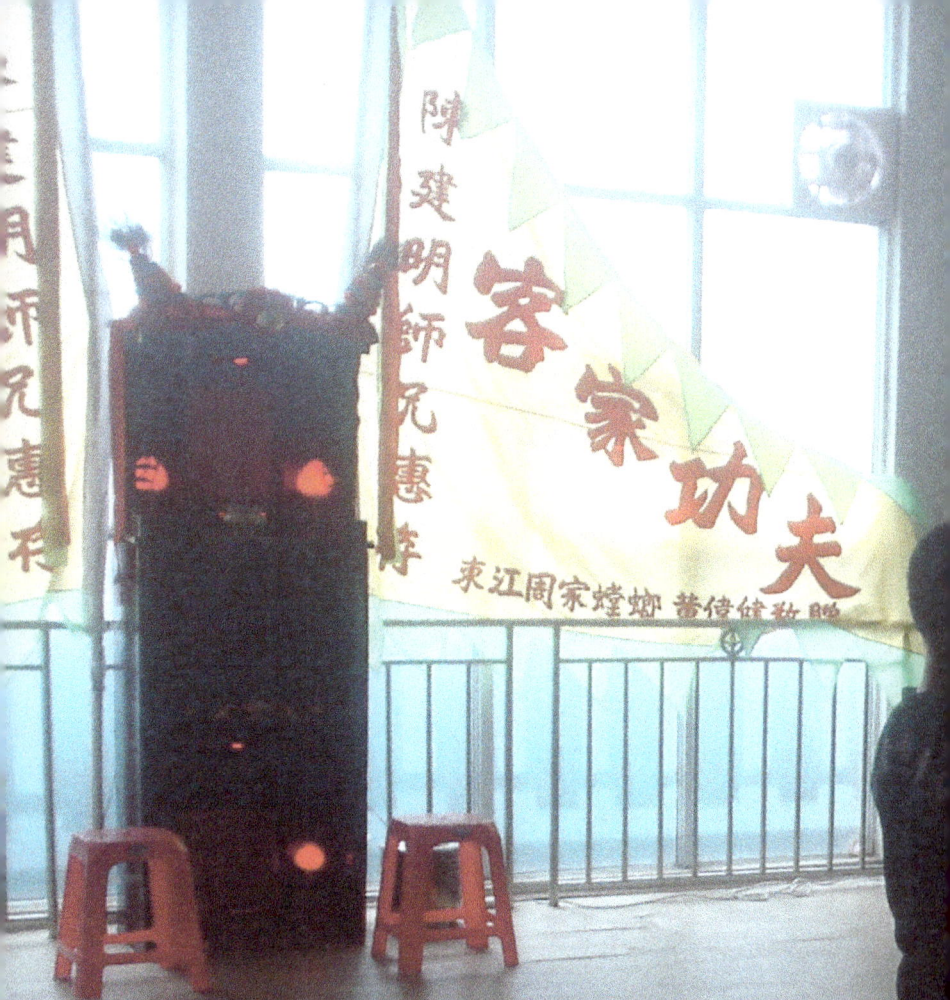

Grandteacher

Lao Siu's

Legacy in China

陳建明師傅
惠州南派螳螂俱樂部

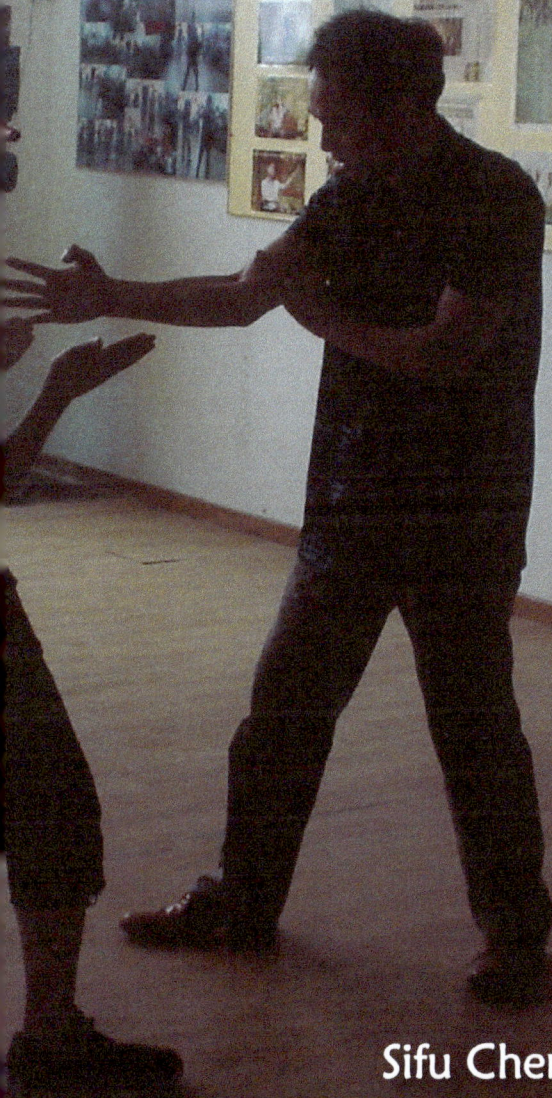

劉水功夫遺產在中國

南螳螂拳師傅陳大師老師

峻学武陳

Sifu Chen Jian Ming, 2014
Huizhou Southern Mantis Boxing School

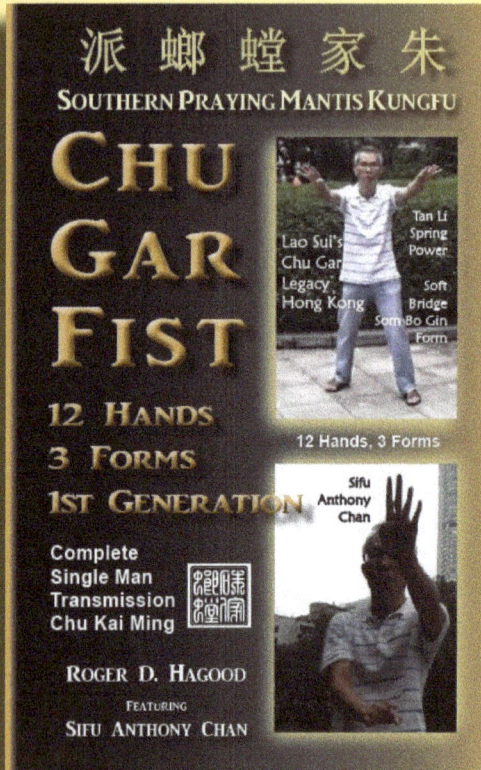
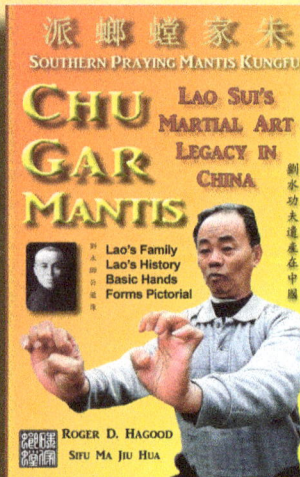
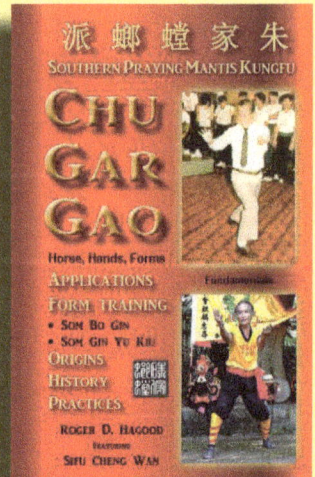

派螂螳家朱

Chu Gar Skills

Wooden Dummy, Yellow Ox Pole, and Dui Jong
Yang Style Chu Gar History and Pictorial

Featuring

Sifu
Yang
Tang Lu

楊譚鹿
師傅

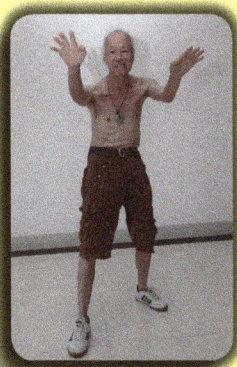

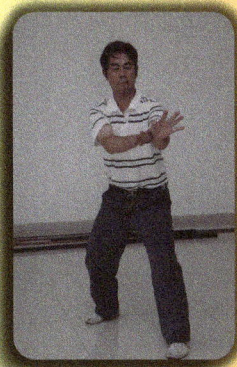

Sifu
Yang
Wei

楊維
師傅

Sifu
Chen
Jian Ming

陳建明
師傅

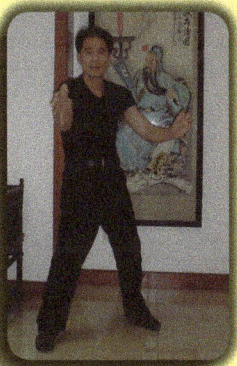

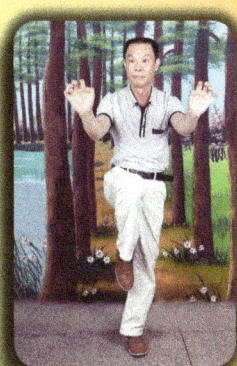

Sifu
Xie
Tian Sheng

谢添胜
師傅

By
Roger D. Hagood

Charles Alan Clemens, Sean W. Robinson, Huang Yan, Editors

Southern Mantis Press | Pingshan Town, China

Southern Mantis Press
5424 NW Cascade Court
Camas, WA 98607
415-359-5077
books@southernmantispress.com

Ordering Information:
Special discounts are available for martial art schools, bookstores, specialty shops, museums and events.   Contact the publisher at the address above.

Cover photograph: Grandmaster Yang Tanglu, Hong Kong, is a descendant of first generation Lao Sui disciple, Yang Shou, from the 1920s. Today the Yang Clan is active in their hometown of Qingxi, Dongguan, China.

ISBN: 978-0-9857240-7-8

Dedication, 獻言

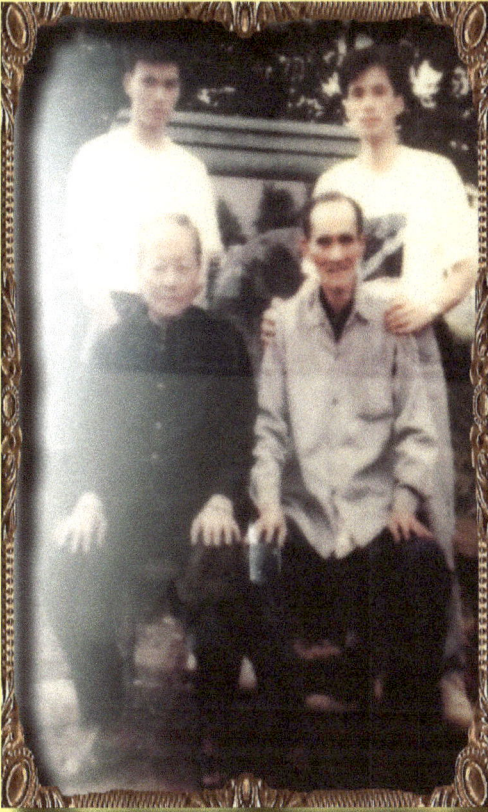

The late Grandmaster Ma Ming Sen and wife seated,
Chen Jianming (standing right), and partner, circa 1972

Sifu Chen Jian Ming, 陳建明 師傅

When Chen Jianming first asked me to cooperate in opening a wuguan together in Lao Sui's hometown he said we should wait until we were sixty years old. At the time, we were both about 56. I thought he probably was just relating to our age by asking and I didn't think about it seriously.

On the third occasion he asked, I took him seriously and after considering the ramifications, I agreed, but said I couldn't be sure I'd be able to walk in another four years and suggested we had

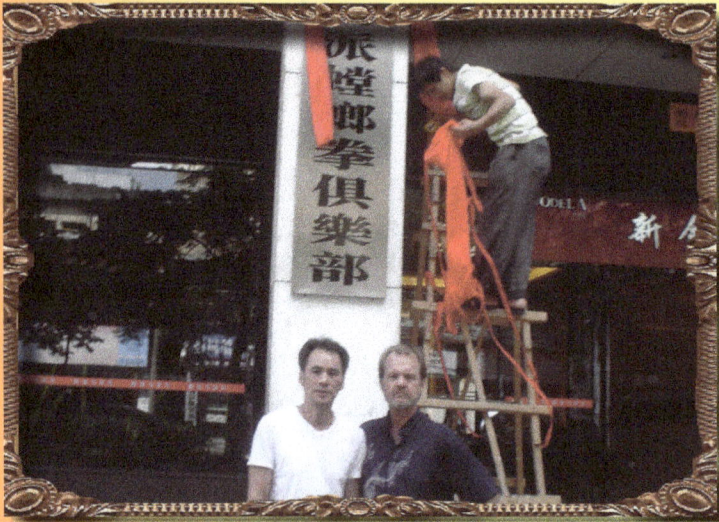

Cheng Jianming (L) and RDH, front and center of the outside billboard placement of the first public Chu Gar School in Lao Sui's hometown.

better do it now.

I had a strong feeling of kinship with Chen Sifu when I first met him (just ask him) and after discovering his martial background and keen interest in Chu Gar Mantis since childhood, I considered the outcome could likely be worth the risk of two tigers on one mountain; two teachers in one School.

Chen Jianming Sifu is an open minded, old fashioned Sifu with a pure pedigree of Chu Gar Mantis. I dedicate this book to his forward thinking and far sighted vision for Chu Gar Mantis' future.

He is much like his own Sifu, Ma Ming Sen, 4th Generation of Chu Gar, in that Chen himself has waited a time with patience, before opening the Chu Gar transmission in Lao Sui's hometown.

I have come to know Chen Jianming Sifu as mentally tough, outwardly rough and inwardly heartfelt - 100% pure Hakka Chinese.

I appreciate him sincerely for inviting me to join him in opening the first Chu Gar School in Lao Sui's hometown and for his brother-friendship. I know his School will blossom after I am gone.

Chen Jianming's Ancestral Shrine
Chu Gar Praying Mantis Kungfu Creed

Hoc Yurn; Hoc Yi; Hoc Kungfu

學仁　學義　學功夫

Jurn Jow; Jurn Si; Jurn Gow Do

尊親　尊師　尊教訓

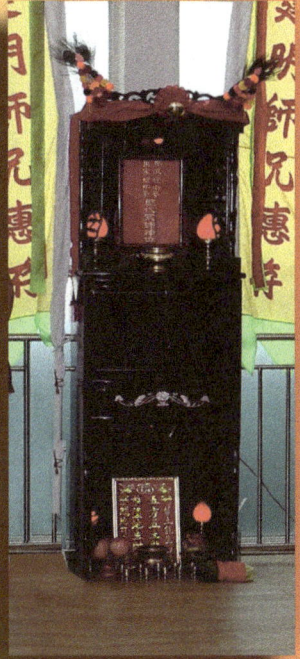

Respect the Ancestors for their transmission of the art.

Respect the Sifu for his teaching.

Respect the Older Brothers for their dedication and loyalty.

Respect the Younger Brothers for determination in training.

Dedication, 獻言

"陈建明第一次邀请我一起在劉水的家乡开一间武馆时说，我们应该等到60岁。当时我们两人都已56岁 。我想他可能只是想问问我的年龄，所以我也没有把它当回事。 当他第三次问起时，我开始认真对待他的话，并在考虑后果之后同意了他的提议。但我说自己不敢保证还能再活四年，并建议我们最好现在开始。 当我第一次见到陈师傅时（只是互相问候了几句），我和他之间就有了一种非常强烈的亲近感。我从小对朱家螳螂充满浓厚的兴趣，并发现他了的武术背景，因此我认为这和一山二虎，一所学校两名教师的危险后果一样。 陈建明师傅是一个思想开放的老派武师，朱家螳螂的直系传人。我谨以此书纪念他对朱家螳螂未来的前瞻性思维和远见卓识。 他很像他的师傅马铭森，朱家螳螂的第四代传人。因为陈师傅在老隋的家乡开朱家螳螂武馆之前总是会耐心地等待。 我所认识的陈建明师傅意志坚韧，外表粗犷，内心真诚 - 100％的纯客家人。 我很感激他能邀请我一起在老隋的家乡开第一间朱家螳螂学校以及与他的兄弟情谊。我知道他的学校一定会在我走后遍地开花。 "

Contents

Contents

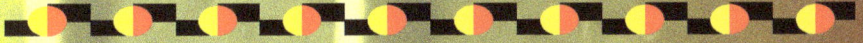

Preface

This book assumes you know and are skillful in the basics of Chu Gar Mantis. You should read my two preceding books on Chu Gar, especially, if you are using this book, as a tutorial. "Don't run the horse before you walk the horse," is a Mantis maxim.

This book is about Sifu Chen Jian Ming and Huizhou City, Guandong, China, Chu Gar Mantis.

Huizhou Chu Gar is pure still. It is second-generation Lao Sui teaching and it is as close to the source, as close to the wellspring, as one can find today. That is because the late Ma Ming Sen went to Hong Kong in 1937, married Lao Sui's adopted daughter, lived and trained with Lao Sui for five years and then returned back to their hometown, Huizhou, in 1941. You see, Ma Ming Sen, from 1941 to 1962, never once mentioned that he was a master of Chu Gar. And you must remember, if you think that five years is not enough for mastery, that even Lao Sui, himself, only trained with his teacher, Wong Fook Go, for four years! (Read my other books.)

Some say it was because of political persecution and later the Cultural Revolution, that Ma kept Lao Sui's teaching to himself, until 1962, when only occasionally he taught his son, Ma Jiuhua, 12 strokes of Chu Mantis boxing. Then, in 1972, Chen Jian Ming, featured in this book, having heard Ma was a Chu Gar teacher, petitioned and became Ma's first disciple. Chen was just a boy of fifteen years then and rode his bicycle three hours to catch the East River boat to Ma's home where he often stayed and trained overnight, in the village, with his teacher. This year Chen is 57 and carries forward this undiluted lineage of Lao Sui's second generation Chu Gar, in their hometown city, Huizhou.

There are other factors at play too. When I say 'undiluted' you should consider the differences in Hong Kong culture, circa 1940, and China proper. Hong Kong was a British colony with a diffusion of International comings and goings. Things were more open than in the mainland. Martial art was no exception and Chu Gar expanded, in the 1950s, as a result of this cultural difference. Many, including Kungfu Sifu, sought haven in Hong Kong for its benefits and so

Preface

martial arts of many styles openly intermingled and proliferated in Hong Kong. This included Lao Sui's teaching and his students, after his passing, in 1942.

As a result, many of Lao Sui's students, in Hong Kong, expanded upon his original teaching, which one could say was quite simple and even primitive with fewer methods. Lao's original Chu Gar method was horse, dui jong, and four forms. After the 1950s, in Hong Kong, Chu Gar Mantis became quite well known for its simple ferocity, all the while, a number of new methods and forms were created.

Therefore, I said, Chen Jian Ming's Huizhou Hakka Mantis, is as close as one can get to Lao Sui's original second generation teaching. And if you are interested in Chu Gar, as a traditional Chinese boxing style, you will do well to study Chen's dummy, pole, and dui jong paired training, in this book.

Yip Sui, in the late 1930's, was also a second generation disciple of Lao's Chu Gar, and a classmate of Ma Ming Sen (the teacher of Chen, featured in this book). It was only Yip, who after Lao Sui passed, who called Lao's teaching 'Chow Gar.' Lao's teaching, in Hong Kong and China today, is still known as Chu Gar. Primarily, it was Yip Sifu who expanded Lao's teaching in the 1950s and later his students added and modified even further, until today, Chow Gar is perhaps more popular than Lao's original Chu Gar teaching. Furthermore, students of Yip Sifu's 'Chow Gar' have today created their own eclectic styles such as "Steel Wire" and "Circular Mantis."

It is honorable to mention that first generation Lao Sui disciples in Shau Kei Wan, Hong Kong, included Yang Shou and Chu Jar Ng (Chu Kai Ming) among others. Their descendents are still teaching in Hong Kong and China today. Watch for their upcoming releases by Southern Mantis Press.

Lest you should think today's Hakka Mantis has lost its early tradition of 'we fix and repair broken kungfu," then let me relate my 2013 experience of joining Chen Jian Ming to open the first public 'wuguan' or martial art School, in Lao Sui's hometown, Huizhou.

Preface

I opened the School every morning for newcomers. Huizhou is an ancient martial art city dating back to 1368. It is the hometown of Southern Long Ying Dragon, White Eyebrow, Li Jia, and other Hakka boxing styles commonly called 'Buddha Fist.' Some visitors who wandered into the new School purposely were not shy in wanting to cross hands. After all, a Mantis maxim states, "If I can pass your hand, why should I learn from you."

On several occasions, I had to apply the Mantis maxim, "give back what you get," sending those who wanted only to test the new School's 'Southern Mantis Boxing' home with a mark. (They used too much power and it was returned back to them.)

And on at least one occasion, Chen Sifu received three visitors who wished to test our Hakka Southern Mantis. One was knocked unconscious and the other two carried him out. Hence, the Mantis maxim, "you don't come, I won't start." They got back what they tried to give.

After all, Hakka Mantis is Chinese boxing. But, in middle age, it is more important to consider tradition, culture, art, and health.

This book will shed light on Lao Sui's original Chu Gar, how to use basic training on a wooden man (or dummy) when a live partner isn't available, the obscure "Yellow Ox Staff' form, and variations of the three original 'dui jong' two man training methods of Lao Sui's Chu Gar Mantis.

It cannot, as a book, teach you. It can only shed light, or more light, depending on the point of your arrival.

RDH
Guangdong, China
Summer, 2015

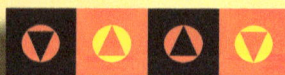

About Chu Gar Mantis Boxing

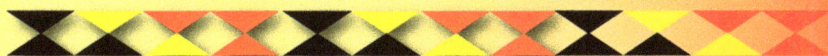

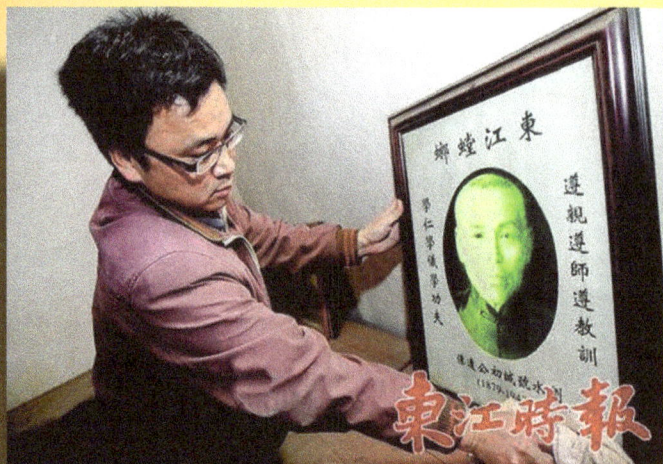

Lao Jian Chang, 38, holds the memorial photograph of his grand uncle Lao Sui, 2013, Huiyang, Huizhou

Chu Gar Mantis School of Lao Sui

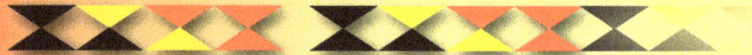

Heng Yuen Village Conceals the Southern School of Mantis Boxing in the Home of Lao Sui

劉水傳朱家螳螂

香園村暗藏南派螳螂拳 ″劉屋洋樓″ 原來有段古

東江流域的民眾自古尚武好義，在惠州產生過東江龍形拳、李家拳、白眉拳等蜚聲中外的拳種，湧現出林耀桂、李義、張禮泉等著名拳師。2月16日，″惠州邊界行″採訪組在蘆洲鎮香園村發現，香園村暗藏一種名叫南派螳螂拳的拳種。仿照螳螂的身形馬步、沉肩墮肘懸吊索三箭拳及吞胸拔背的筲箕背鐵尺腰......剛柔並濟的螳螂拳，讓人大飽眼福。

16

Since ancient times, the people of the Dongjiang East River basin have been skilled in warfare. In Huizhou City, there is the Dongjiang Dragon Fist boxing, Li Gar, and White Eyebrow boxing, which emerged from the famous masters named Lin Yaogui, Li Yi, and Zhang Liquan. On February 16, 2012, an interview by the East River Times Newspaper found a hidden faction of Southern Mantis boxing in Luchou Town, Hong Yuen Village. Modeled on a mantis' movements, boxers learn firm steps, soft and hard power, sink the chest and round the back, iron waist, and Three Step Arrow boxing. It is a feast for the eyes.

The Southern Mantis School third-generation descendant, Lao Sui, flourished in Hong Kong in the 1930s. However, as recently as 2008, the disciples and family members of Lao Sui in Huizhou, China, Lao's hometown, discovered that by accident Southern Praying Mantis in Hong Kong had divided into two factions, Chow Gar and Chu Gar. Accordingly, further research was conducted in the location where this Southern Mantis originated, Meizhou, China. It was discovered that Chow and Chu pronunciation in Meizhou Hakka dialect are very similar, but the original ancestor in China is named Chu (Zhu) Ya Nan. Chu's descendants still live in this area. Without question, the name of Lao Sui's Mantis legacy in China and his hometown is Chu Gar from Chu Ya Nan.

However, to avoid confusion we can say that the whole of Southern Mantis may be collectively referred to today as Dongjiang (East River) Southern Praying Mantis without the distinction of Chow or Chu.

Lao Sui trains Chu Gar four years under his Master, Wong Fook Go

Today in Luchou Town, Hong Yuen Village, remains a two story brick and wood home that was built by Lao Sui circa 1936. The second floor has a large balcony with peaches, bats, and other sculptures on thick wooden eaves which are engraved with auspicious Chinese words like "lucky." The double door main entrance is still solid and steady. There is a story of the martial artist, Lao Sui, behind this old building which is still the family home of his descendants today. (Refer to page 143.)

17

南派螳螂拳第三代傳人劉水將該拳種在香港發揚光大。不過，讓南派螳螂拳惠州弟子們意外的是，該拳種在香港有周家和朱家兩派之分。據他們前往五華縣轉水鎮蓮塘村考證，周和朱兩字在梅州客家話中極為相似，南派螳螂拳的宗師應為朱亞南。他們因此計畫為南派螳螂拳正名，取消周、朱之分，統稱為南派東江螳螂拳。

劉水20歲拜師學螳螂拳24歲赴港開館授徒

據香港出版的拳譜、劉水弟子葉瑞編寫的《東江螳螂拳》記載，時際清末，劉水避亂至香港，因技高德偉，遐邇知名，桃李遍港九，從學者無數。

在蘆洲鎮香園村，有一棟民國時期的兩層磚木結構小洋樓，二樓有寬大的陽臺，翹角的屋簷上有壽桃、蝙蝠等雕塑點綴，還刻有"吉祥"、"如意"等字樣，條石砌成的大門顯得堅實、沉穩。這棟樓被當地人稱為"劉屋洋樓"，在舊屋原址上修建，已有70年曆史，背後隱藏著一位武術家的故事。

這位武術家的名字叫劉水，號初誠，1879年生於香園村。劉水自幼愛好無數，年少時習馬家拳，還自創了劉水棍術，20歲時已以拳棍聞名鄉里。蘆洲與觀音閣隔著東江相望，當時，蘆洲人常乘船到觀音閣鎮趁圩。每到觀音閣鎮圩日，劉水喜歡去逛一逛，尋找高手比武。

彼時，南派螳螂拳第二代傳人、興甯人黃福高適逢到觀音閣行醫賣藥，見劉水是一個習武的好苗子，就對劉水說他的功夫很好，可惜還未到上乘之境。年少氣盛的劉水要求與黃福高比武。幾個回合下來，劉水就被黃福高制伏。劉水當即跪拜黃福高為師，跟著師傅學南派螳螂拳，當時劉水只有20歲。

經過黃福高4年的精心指導，劉水練就一身過硬的南派螳螂拳，還學會了刀槍、跌打醫術，成為南派螳螂拳第三代傳人。1903年，24歲的劉水到香港發展，在香港九龍開館授徒。據香港出版的拳譜、劉水弟子葉瑞編寫的《東江螳螂拳》記載，時際清末，劉水避亂至香港，因技高德偉，遐邇知名，桃李遍港九，從學者無數。

18

Lao Sui's original name was Lao Cheng and he was born in 1879, in the aforementioned Hong Yuen Village. Since childhood Lao had a love of martial arts and trained all kinds of local Hakka kungfu. By the age of 20, he was quite famous for his staff skills and readily taught others boxing. Just across the East River was the Goddess of Mercy Pavilion (Guanyinge) and the Luchou people often crossed over by boat on their way to the market. On festive days, Lao Sui would go around seeking martial art masters to have a contest.

On one such occasion, the second generation Southern Mantis descendant, Wong Fook Go from Xingning City, happened to be at the Goddess of Mercy Pavilion practicing medicine and selling drugs. There he observed Lao Sui's kungfu but said that it appeared good but wasn't really useful. And so, the young and fit Lao Sui engaged Wong in several rounds of boxing, each of which Lao was easily subdued. Immediately Lao recognized Wong had superior skill and kowtowed to become Wong Fook Go's pupil when he was 20 years old.

After four years of careful guidance, Lao Sui had become an excellent Southern Mantis boxer and also had learned the skills of knives and guns, bone setting, and medicine and became known as the third-generation descendant of Chu Gar Southern Praying Mantis. In 1903, the 24 year old Lao went to Hong Kong and never returned to his birthplace.

Lao Sui Builds a Home But Does Not Return to His Roots

In 1936 Lao Sui was over the age of 50, and had the idea of returning to his roots. So he asked a friend to bring money back to Huizhou to build a home. It took more than four years to complete construction. Today, his family still lives in this house.

After arriving in Hong Kong, Lao Sui taught Chu Gar boxing and his younger brother, Lao Fu Yuan studied medicine. After Fu Yuan completed his study, he went back to their family home in Luchou and passed down his knowledge to his family. In 2013, Lao Jian Chang, the grandson of Lao Fu Yuan, has inherited the mantle and continues practicing medicine in the home Lao Sui had constructed in 1936.

建"劉屋洋樓"無奈落葉難歸根

劉屋洋樓"建于1936年，當時劉水年逾50，有落葉歸根的想法，當時在香港托朋友帶錢回來。這房子一建就是4年多。

雖然劉水離開家鄉，但對故鄉蘆洲的思念及與親友的聯繫交往卻從未斷絕。

劉水在香港設館教拳師，他的弟弟劉富元曾到香港跟其學醫，得其真傳，後回到觀音閣、蘆洲等地，成為一代名醫。而今，劉富元的孫子劉振強繼承其衣缽，繼續在香園村行醫，繼續居住在"劉屋洋樓"裡。

"劉屋洋樓"建于1936年，當時劉水年逾50，有葉落歸根的想法，當時在香港托朋友帶錢回來。這房子一建就是4年多，1941年竣工時，日軍已全面入侵中國，香港淪陷。

劉水曾經返回家鄉，但回至深圳時身體不適，又因為戰亂交通阻塞，只好折返香港。劉水遺留下來的兩首詩，一首可以看出他當時的思鄉之情："虛度光陰數十年，今春首采假居先；歸家心急如星火，斷絕交通恨不前；欲圖冒險回桑梓，中途兵災又掛牽；雖是暫時羈此地，誠驚故我亦依然。"

另一首則看出劉水歸鄉無望後的失望之情："浪跡江湖覓食多，平生志願望蹉跎；香園歸隱非吾願，六親情切付東河。大地既無干淨土，宗邦禦敵動干戈。從今勘破紅塵界，萬念皆空一夢柯。"

思鄉心切的劉水，積慮于心，1942年在香港抱憾去世，享年64歲，離鄉30載未歸，魂散香江。

弟子馬銘森在惠收徒傳授螳螂拳
馬銘森稱呼劉水為"同年爺"。1937年，30歲的馬銘森到香港拜劉水學武，一學就是5年，練就一身功夫，並于1941年返鄉。

雖然劉水沒有在惠州教授過弟子，但因為香園村人馬銘森

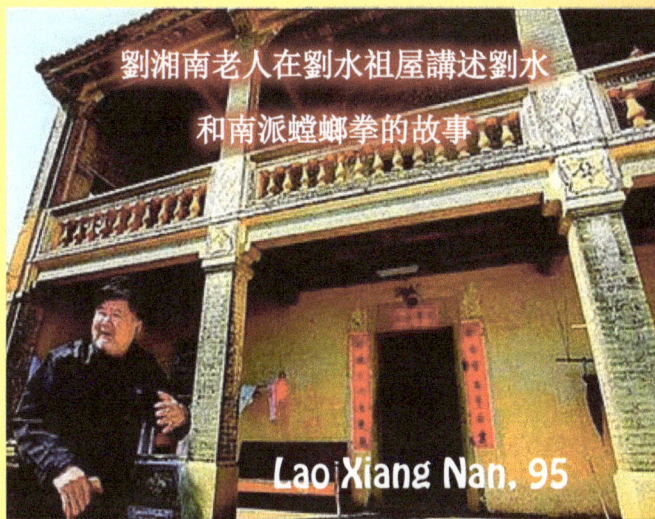

劉湘南老人在劉水祖屋講述劉水
和南派螳螂拳的故事

Lao Xiang Nan, 95

Lao Xiang Nan, 95, plays Chu Gar Mantis at the home Lao Sui financed but never was able to see. Lao Xiang Nan is the son of Lao Fu Yuan, Lao Sui's brother.

Once, Lao Sui decided to return home but upon reaching Shenzhen, just inside China's border, could not go further due to the Japanese invading China. Travelling wasn't easy and Lao's health had also taken a turn for the worse. Although within days of reaching his home, he decided to turn back to Hong Kong.

Later on he wrote some lines of poetry expressing his feelings of being homesick. (Refer to the translations on page 156 - 157.) Lao actively kept his family in mind until his passing in 1942, at age 64. He was never able to return home. His final resting place is in Hong Kong today.

Disciple Ma Ming Sen Returns Chu Gar Mantis to Huizhou

In Lao Sui's village, the Ma family was the Lao family's next door neighbor. The Ma and Lao families still live next door to each other in 2013. Their families are related by marriage as well. It was Ma Ming Sen who married Lao Sui's daughter. In 1937, the 30 year old Ma Ming Sen went to Hong Kong to learn Southern Mantis from Lao Sui. There he trained five years before returning back to their hometown, Huiyang, in 1941.

Lao Sui left for Hong Kong in 1903 and never returned to his hometown in China. It is because of his Son-in-law, Ma Ming Sen,

赴港學武，使得南派螳螂拳得以在惠州傳承。

據馬銘森的兒子、今年71歲的馬九華介紹，他的祖父與劉水是同齡結拜兄弟，馬銘森稱呼劉水為"同年爺"。1937年，30歲的馬銘森到香港拜劉水學武，一學就是5年，練就一身功夫，並于1941年返鄉。

令人疑惑的是，馬銘森在回來的二三十年間，幾乎沒有向外人展露過武功。"父親回鄉後，歷經抗戰和解放戰爭，建國後又歷經特殊的政治環境，這也許是他未展露武功的根源。"馬九華說，到1962年，他21歲的時候，馬銘森才偶爾教他一兩招螳螂拳鍛煉身體。

直至陳建明出現，馬銘森身懷絕技的秘密才被大家所知。1957年出生的陳建明，從小就喜歡舞刀弄槍，其父親當時在蘆洲鎮供銷社工作，打聽到馬銘森會功夫。1972年，陳建明拜馬銘森為師。後來，馬銘森在蘆洲鎮以及觀音閣鎮一帶也收了一些徒弟，觀音閣鎮人謝添勝就是其中之一。馬銘森每到觀音閣鎮時，都會到謝添勝家教他打拳。

1984年，77歲的馬銘森應邀到水口的一家武館當師傅，收了70多個徒弟，但真正學成者極少。1996年，90歲高齡的馬銘森在故里去世。

馬九華說，馬銘森屬於南派螳螂拳第四代傳人，該拳在惠弟子基本師承馬銘森。

惠州第子去五華縣轉水鎮蓮塘村考證祖師爺姓名

馬九華、謝添勝等人去興甯五華縣朱亞南老家考證，證實朱家教創始人是朱亞南、不是周亞南、所以劉水宗師傳受下來的應是朱家螳螂。

近些年，隨著武術運動的勃興，各種拳派尋根問祖熱也在興起。"劉屋洋樓"曾接待來自五湖四海的南派螳螂拳弟子，這些弟子們，均尊稱劉水為"一代宗師"。

與此同時，南派螳螂拳在惠州的傳人，也開始了尋根之

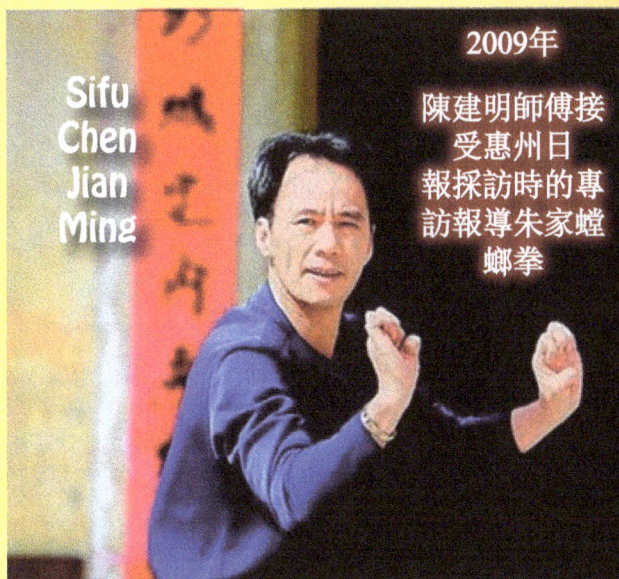

2009年

陳建明師傅接
受惠州日
報採訪時的專
訪報導朱家螳
螂拳

Sifu Chen Jian Ming

Chen Jian Ming, 55, is a leader of Chu Gar Mantis in Lao Sui's hometown today. He is the chief pupil of Lao Sui's Son-in-law, Ma Ming Sen.

that Chu Gar exists in Lao Sui's hometown today.

According to Ma Ming Sen's son, 71 year old Ma Jiuhua (cover of this book), his grandfather and Lao Sui, being village neighbors, were sworn brothers of the same age.

Ma Jiuhua said it was puzzling that for some years after returning from Hong Kong, his father, Ma Ming Sen, never showed or talked about learning Chu Gar Mantis from Lao Sui. It was the time of the Anti-Japanese War and the War of Liberation, and a special political environment existed, so perhaps the elder Ma did not expose his martial art for fear of persecution. Ma Jiuhua states that in 1962, when he was 21 years old, his father Ma Ming Sen only occasionally taught him twelve strokes Mantis boxing workouts.

Until Chen Jianming appeared in 1972, it was a great secret, in Lao Sui's home village, that Ma Ming Sen was a master of Chu Gar Mantis Kungfu. Chen Jianming was born in 1957, and his family was from Luchou town. As a boy, Chen trained Li Gar, Dragon and many kinds of village boxing. By accident he overheard a friend of his father talking about Ma Ming Sen's Chu Gar Mantis and so he travelled the long distance by small boat on the East River to ask Ma Ming Sen to teach him. Ma refused. Persistent, Chen returned many times by riding a bicycle more than 3 hours each time to petition Ma Sifu. Each time Ma refused. But one day, Ma spotted the young Chen Jian Ming playing kungfu and recognized

旅。2008年，馬九華等10多名師兄弟前往香港九龍拜會劉水嫡傳弟子葉瑞、鄭運等人。不過，讓馬九華等人困惑的是，在香港，由劉水發揚光大的南派螳螂拳都冠以 "東江" 之名，但卻分為周家和朱家兩拳派。

馬九華估計，這應該不是劉水弟子故意另立門戶，而可能是音誤。按照粵語發音，周和朱兩字發言極易分別，但五華客家話中的周和朱讀音難以辨別，基本是同一種讀音。馬九華認為，南派螳螂拳前三代均是客家人，有可能將周和朱混淆並傳播，造成了今日的分歧。按照葉瑞的資訊，南派螳螂拳的創始人應為周亞南，廣東興甯周家村人；而按照鄭運的理解，應為朱亞南，廣東五華人。到底孰對孰錯？

去年11月，馬九華等人前往五華興甯，遍尋興甯也找不到周家村。後來，他們又到了梅州五華，在五華轉水鎮蓮塘村找到了朱亞南的身份資訊和習拳經歷。

原來，朱亞南正是南派螳螂拳的祖師爺，于清朝中葉、200多年前到福建南少林追隨禪隱大師學習南少林拳，目睹螳螂與雀相鬥，創出螳螂拳。為了區別北方的螳螂拳，遂將其命名為南派螳螂拳。出寺後，朱亞南到東江一帶傳授給客家弟子，黃福高便是其一。

為了證明亞南姓 "朱" 而非 "周"，南派螳螂拳在興甯的第四傳人范金茂去年11月29日寫字條給馬九華，稱只有五華縣轉水鎮蓮塘村朱亞南，興甯市沒有周家村，沒有周亞南，如有不詳細者可到興甯、五華來調查。

南派螳螂拳祖師爺的名字終於水落石出，馬九華如釋重負。他把這些考究成果都展覽在他自己設立的香園村南派螳螂拳陳列館裡。他和其他師兄弟都希望為南派螳螂拳正名：興甯五華沒有周家螳螂拳派，南派螳螂拳應姓朱。他們希望早日將這個誤差告知香港的拳師們。

因為南派螳螂拳一開始是在東江一帶傳承，在揚名之地香港，該拳也被叫做東江螳螂拳，馬九華希望，能將此拳統稱為南派東江螳螂拳，並世代在東江一帶傳承下去。

that he had a great talent for martial arts. Thereafter, he agreed to teach Chen and from 1972 until Ma Ming Sen's passing in 1996 they enjoyed a strong familial teacher-student relationship.

Chen states that Ma Sifu usually taught him from 9pm until 2 or 3 in the morning hours. And that he often would continue to self-train until day break. Some years later, in the vicinity of Luchou town and the Goddess of Mercy Pavilion, Ma Sifu accepted 3 other pupils including Xie Tian Sheng. Today, Chen and Xie continue teaching Chu Gar Mantis in Lao's hometown area.

In 1984, the 77 year old Ma Ming Sen was invited to teach Chu Gar Mantis in nearby Sui Ko Town. There was a large martial arts Association with more than 70 apprentices all by the surname, Yan. Even though Ma taught them, he stated there were very few who really studied.

In 1996, the 90 year old Ma Ming Sen died in his hometown. It is said he stayed up very late until after 5 am, as was his custom, chatting around with all his family as usual, until he said he felt a bit tired and retired. Early the next morning around 6 am, it was discovered he had passed peacefully in his bed.

Ma Ming Sen was the fourth-generation descendant of Chu Gar Mantis in China. He was a disciple of Lao Sui as well as his Son-in-law. Today the Lao and Ma families are still living in the same locations as nearly 100 years before.

Huizhou Disciples go to Meizhou to Research Chu Gar's Patron Deity

Ma Jiuhua Sifu and the others would like to inform all fellow boxers that in China, the legacy of Lao Sui is Chu Gar Mantis and the teaching is descended from ancestor Chu Ya Nan. There is no Chow Gar faction.

In recent years, Southern Mantis has emerged to the public's attention and in the martial arts community many people have known Lao Sui as a great master. Some foreigners have found their way to Lao Sui's hometown to pay respect.

At the same time, the descendants of Chu Gar Mantis in China began a tour to find its deepest roots. In 2008, Ma Jiuhua and over 10 teacher brothers travelled to Hong Kong, Kowloon, and called on the disciples of Lao Sui, including those of Yip Sui and Cheng Wan. However, Ma Jiuhua and all were puzzled that although Lao Sui's Southern Praying Mantis had flourished in Hong Kong as "East River Mantis," it was yet divided into the Chow and Chu factions.

The China descendants of Lao Sui reasoned this error likely occurred because of the Cantonese and Hakka difference in pronunciation. The Chow faction of Lao Sui's disciple, Yip Sui, stated that Zhou Ya Nan was an ancestor of Zhou family village in Xingning; the Chu disciples of Lao Sui in Hong Kong stated that Chu Ya Nan is ancestor.

Chow or Chu family surname
Chow Gar = Chu Gar
Chow = Zhou (Pinyin)
Chu = Zhu (Pinyin)
Gar = Jia (family)
Gao = Jiao (creed)

And so, Ma Jiuhua and the brothers travelled to Meizhou and Xingning, and nowhere could be found a Chow family village or Chow Ya Nan ancestor. However, in Meizhou, Wuhua, Zhuan Shui Zhen, Liantang Village, Chu Ya Nan's identity and boxing was known and identified by the name Chu Gar Gao and Chu Gar Mantis. In China, the Southern Mantis boxing of Wong Fook Go and Lao Sui is Chu Gar Mantis.

Chu Ya Nan is precisely the patron deity of Chu Gar Southern Praying Mantis. In the Ching dynasty, Chu travelled to the Southern Shaolin Temple in Fujian where he followed a Zen monk who had mastered Southern Shaolin boxing. Chu there witnessed a praying mantis eating a bird and from this, in secret, created the boxing that became known as Chu Gar or Chu family, using his own surname, Chu. Later the Zen monk and Chu combined skills.

In order to distinguish between the Northern Mantis boxing, the name of Southern Praying Mantis was attached. Chu Ya Nan later travelled down the East River area to teach to Hakka disciples, and

among them was Wong Fook
Go, a wandering medicine
seller, who taught Lao Sui.
(Note: In 2013, Chu Ya Nan's
grandson, several generations
down the line, still lives in
Boluo, nearby Lao Sui's village
home.)

In Xingning, from whence
2nd generation, Wong Fook
Go, came, 4th generation
descendant, elder Fan Jinmao,
has written to Ma Jiuhua, to
state that in the area where
this boxing originated there
is only Chu Gar from Chu Ya
Nan. There can be found no
Chow or Chow Ya Nan. Elder
Fan encouraged anyone to
come there to investigate for
themselves.

And so, today in Lao Sui's
village, is a small gallery
established by Ma Jiuhua and
the others, in honor of Lao
Sui's Chu Gar Mantis legacy in
China. It is hoped the world
over will appreciate Chu Gar
Mantis as descended from Chu
Ya Nan and passed down five
or six generations now. As
this boxing school originated
along the Guangdong East
River, it is the hope of Lao
Sui's disciples in China that
all may simply refer to it as
"East River Southern Praying
Mantis." (©今日惠州网，天鹅城
网 Excerpted from Dongjiang
Times Newspaper ### End)

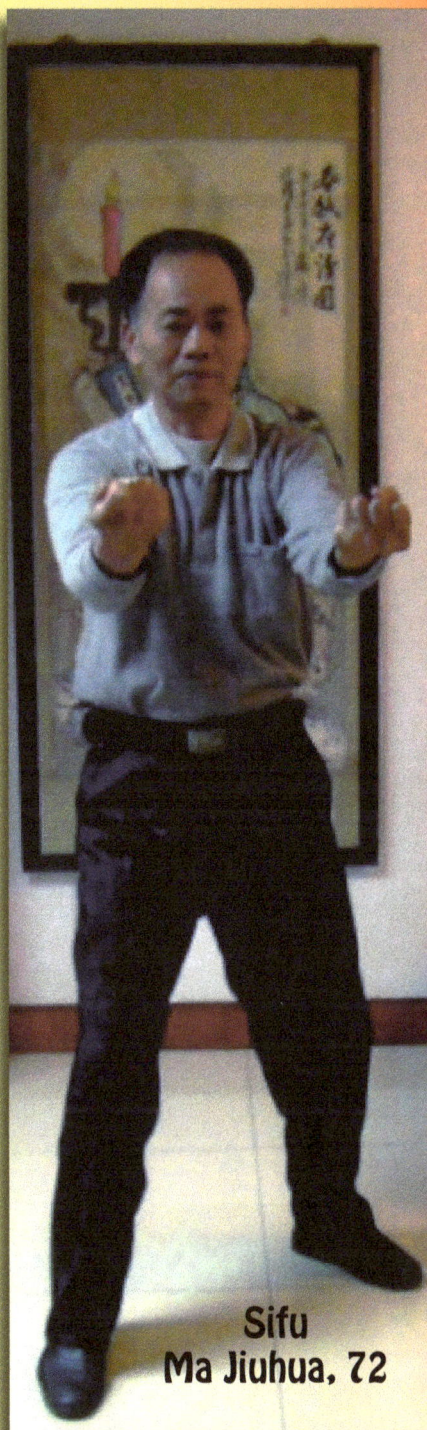

Sifu
Ma Jiuhua, 72

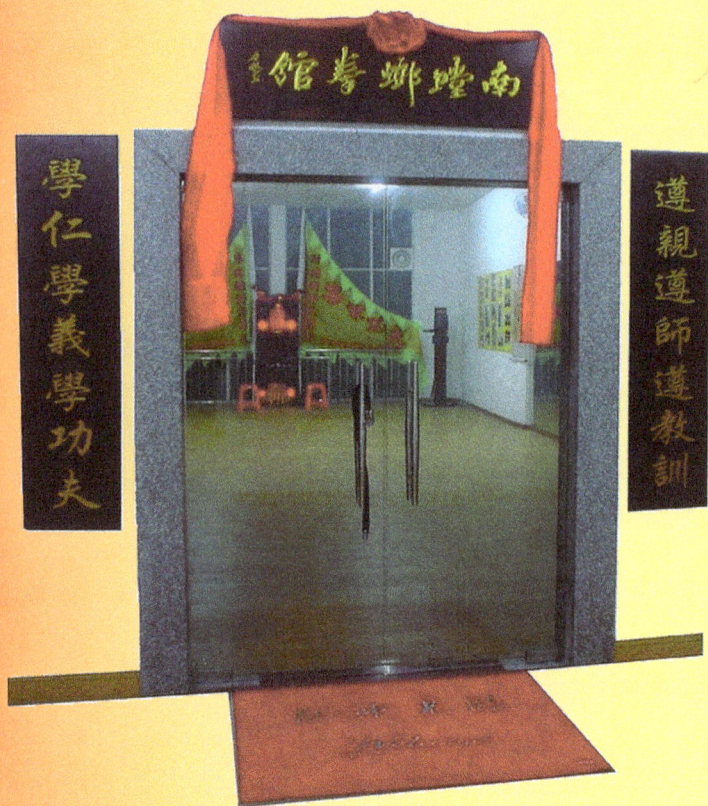

2013 年朱家歷史事件

第一個朱家武館在劉師父的家鄉開幕

有些人把朱家在劉師父家鄉的第一個公眾武館的開幕比喻為一件歷史事件。這比喻是正確的，至少有兩個原因。 並非最不重要的是，我，這本書的作者，RDH，一個非中國人，被邀請參與這新武館的開幕和教學。

其次，這家歷史性的活動匯集了三個源流的朱家一起合作。其中有來自惠州的劉水源流的陳建明師父。 陳建明師父開了自己的新的武館。楊壽-楊維師父，葉瑞源流周家李天來。這三個派別參加都參加在劉水師父故鄉第一個公眾朱家學校的開幕。那麼，第四個原因，因為我（RDH），是鄭運師父朱家香港協會委任的主席。

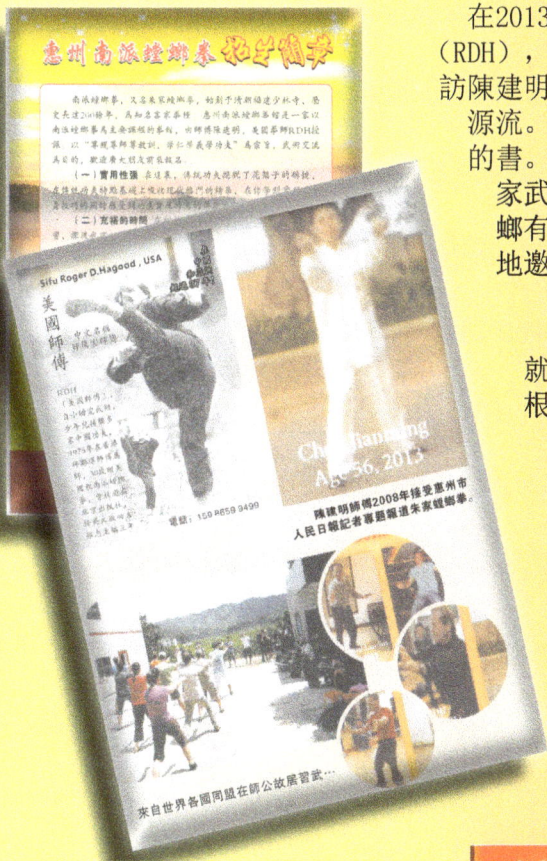

來自世界各國同道在師公故居展習武…

在2013年的最初幾個月，我，（RDH），前往劉水師父的故鄉拜訪陳建明師父和拜訪劉水師父的源流。我們一起合作寫作以下的書。陳師父想開設第一個朱家武館。因為知道我對南螳螂有強大的背景和興趣，特地邀請我參與他的學校的開幕和教學合作。

就這樣，計劃開始了，並根據當地的風水師的吉祥徵兆挑選吉祥的開幕日期和時間！請繼續閱讀以知道了更多關於這家歷史悠久的學校。

以上：關於武館開幕的傳單，內有陳建明師父和RDH的簡歷和有關學校的詳細好處和上課時間，以及一些朱家歷史。

右邊：劉水功夫遺產在中國系列的第一本書，內詳敘劉水師父的家庭背景，歷史，以及朱家基本拳擊的兩個套路。以後的書將會包括（Yellow Ox Tongue Staff）以及四門驚勁.

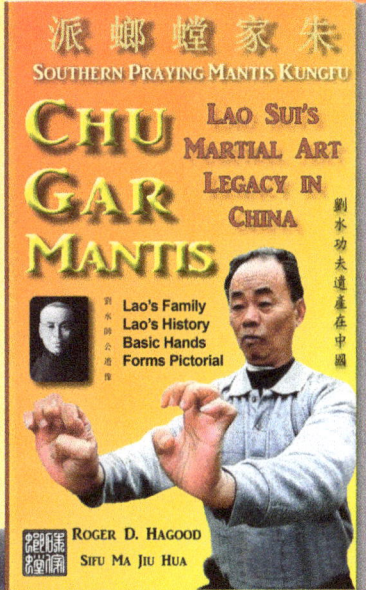

經過了兩個月的準備，終於在7月1日上午9點盛大開幕。在這過去短短的期間有很多事情處理。

從確保符合當局法律，在一個空的建築設計，創建學院，邀請嘉賓和安排他們的住宿，兩個月是相對較短的時間。更何況，我們還親訪 Yang Wei 師父，並要求他的麒麟藝術團進行隆重開幕儀式。

邊欄：惠州是上古門派的城發源地，記錄遠及公元800年。在此發源的門派包括龍，白眉。這兩位創始人的老家園依然保持在這新朱家學校的附近。此外，還有許多客家源流，如李家，李家教，佛手和其他目前還在當地流傳的源流。然而，大部分的舊傳統已被跆拳道甚至 MMA取代。

陳建明師傅
惠州南派螳螂俱樂部

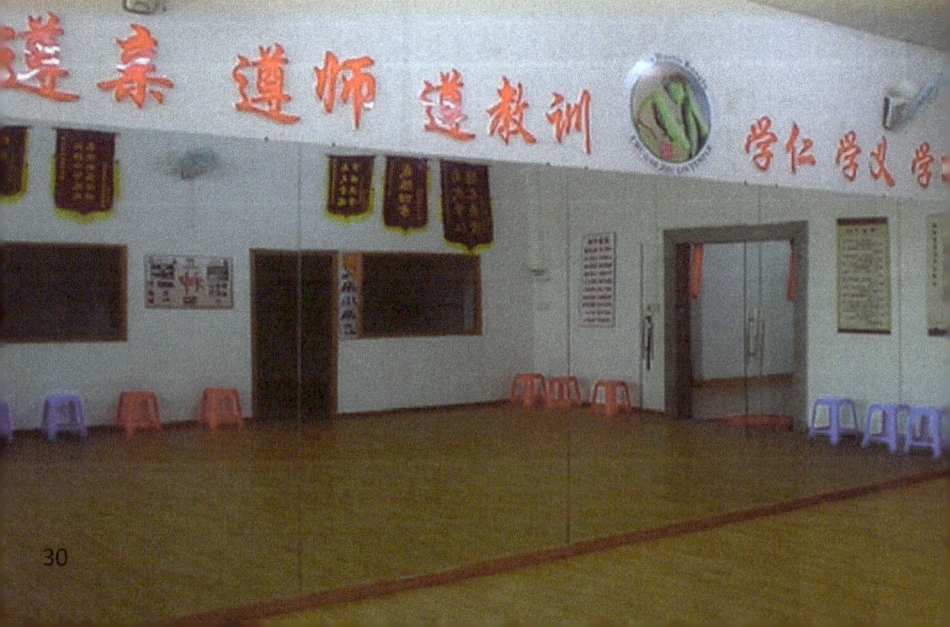

Yang Wei 師父是楊壽的後代。楊壽是劉水師父早期在香港的學生之一。楊壽頗負盛名。

甚至有些人說，他本人可能是第三代朱家傳人。

今天，靠近廣州，在廣東省的首府，Yang Wei 和楊氏族盛大的保持著客家朱家拳擊的傳統。他們還積極參與舞麒麟的傳統和比賽。

因此，Yang Wei，他的團隊約有15名成員被邀請到這裡來，為朱家在劉水師父故鄉的新學校開幕。
他是嘉賓名單中的首要人物。嘉賓名單中包括許多尊敬的師父，來自當地的客家團體，惠州當地政府武術協會和來自香港的葉瑞源流周家螳螂李天來師父。

Sifu Chen Jian Ming
Huizhou Southern Mantis Boxing School

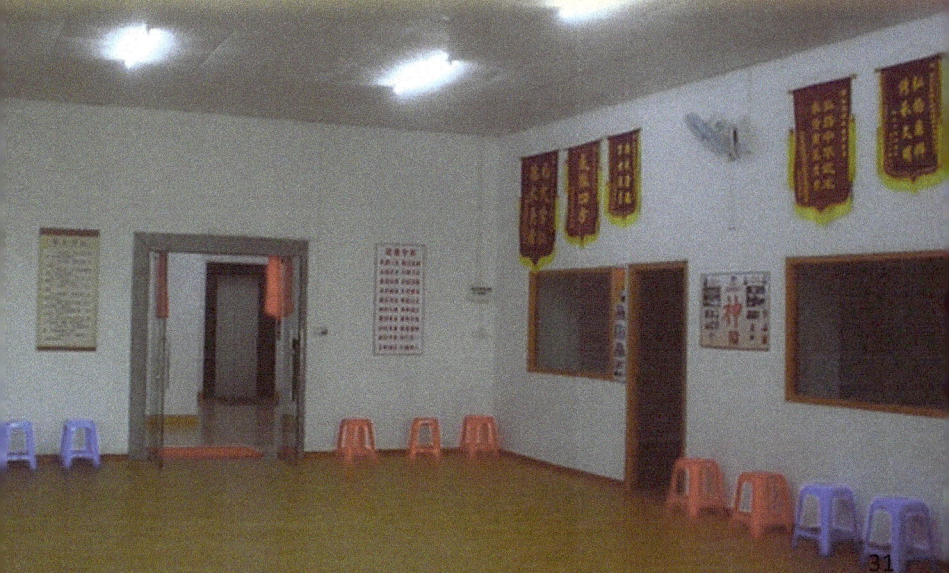

以上：在兩個學校的歷史和世系圖表列出劉水遺留在中國大陸和香港：劉水第三代，馬銘森第四代，陳建明第五代，和RDH第六代在其中。照片顯示，劉水和馬銘森。

下面：Yang Wei 師父的朱家麒麟家族進行盛大的開幕式和呈獻橫幅給陳建明及RDH。

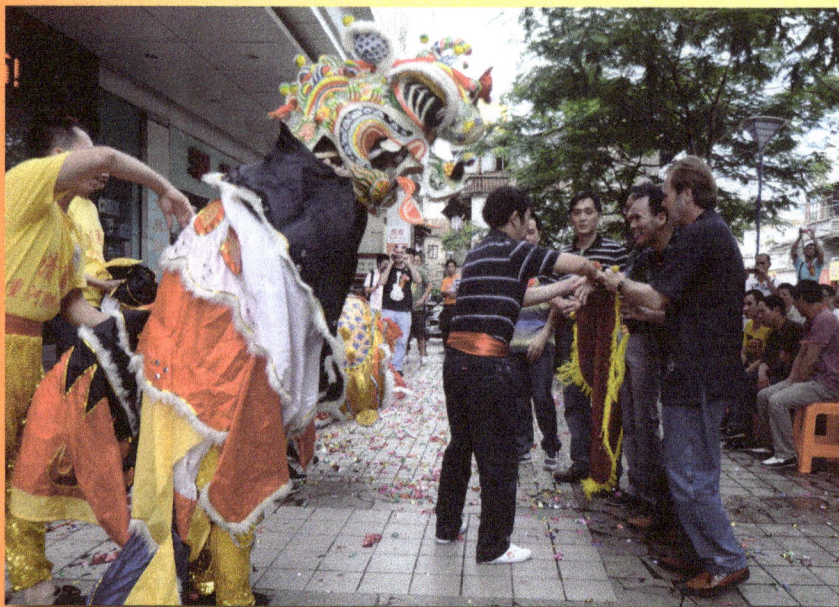

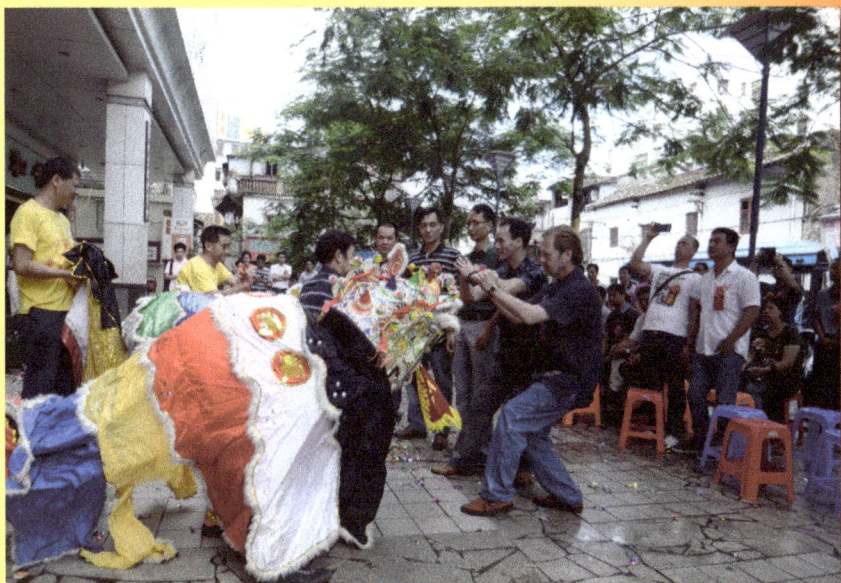

以上：陈建明和RDH向Yang Wei师父的麒麟回敬礼，當地官員在看著。

以下：學校祖堂掛著客家功夫和南派螳螂的黃旗。黃色的旗是李天來香港周家派送的。 左側壁的歷史圖表上顯示 葉瑞和李師父。

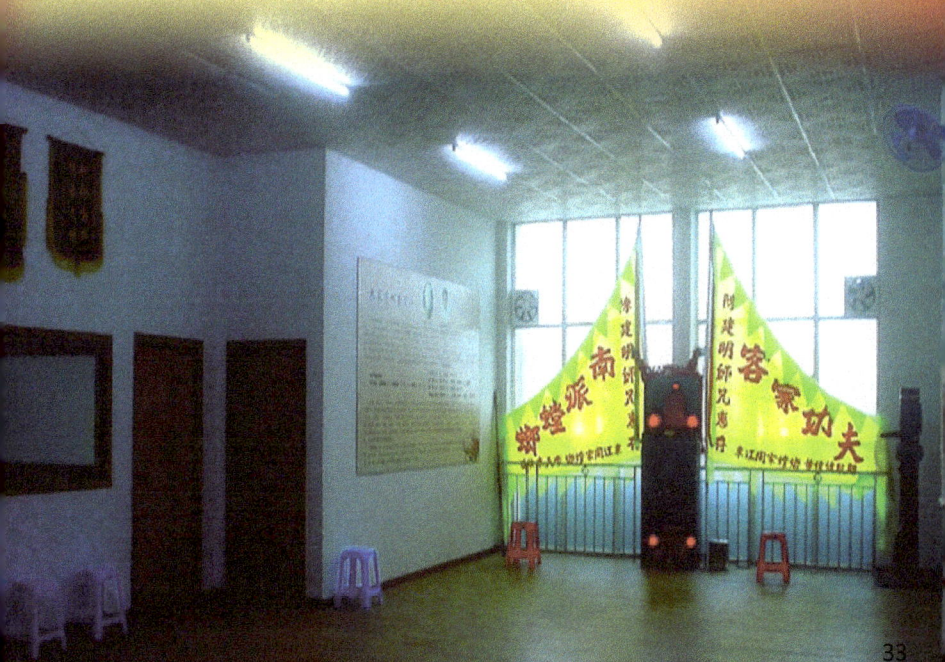

惠州南派螳螂俱樂部

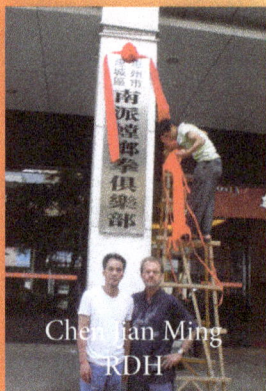

Chen Jian Ming RDH

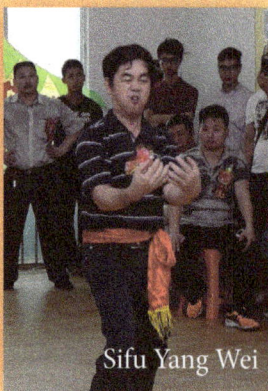

Sifu Yang Wei

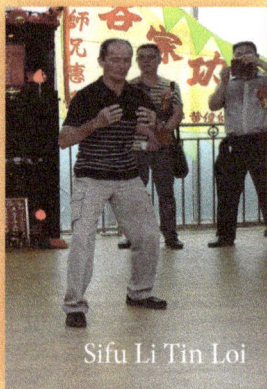

Sifu Li Tin Loi

2013年7月1日盛大的開幕

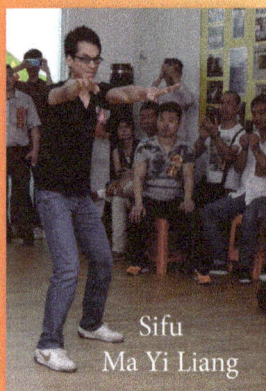

Sifu Ma Yi Liang

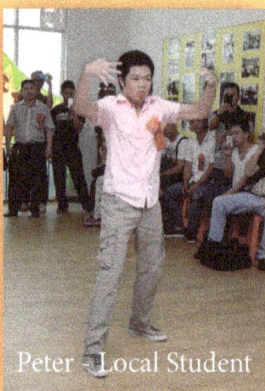

Peter - Local Student

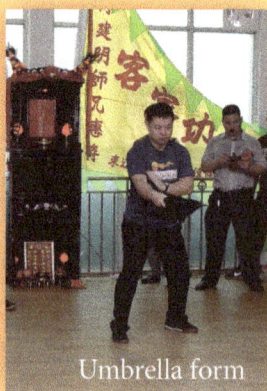

Umbrella form

劉水朱家螳螂遺產在中國

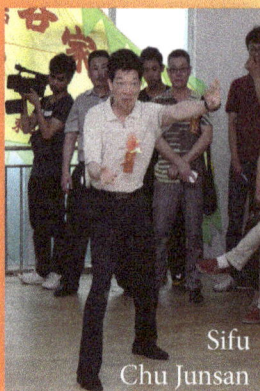

Sifu Chu Junsan

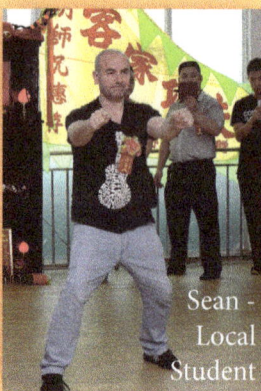

Sean - Local Student

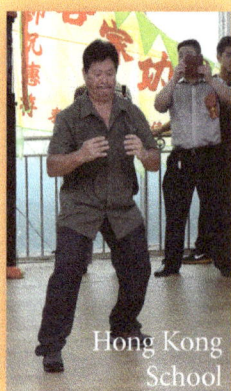

Hong Kong School

陳建明師父的朱家學校，在惠城，惠州，廣東，中國

34

Huizhou Southern Mantis Boxing School

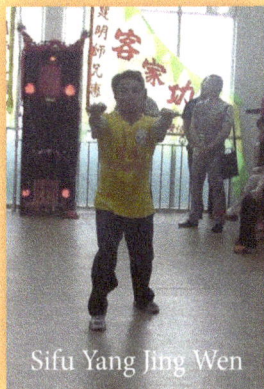

Sifu Yang Jing Wen

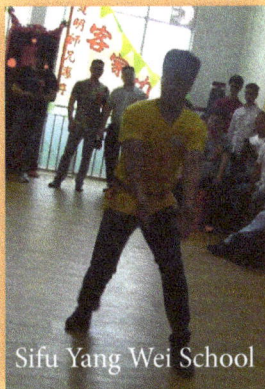

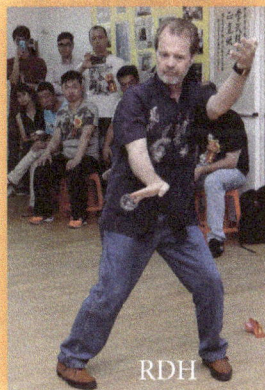

Sifu Yang Wei School

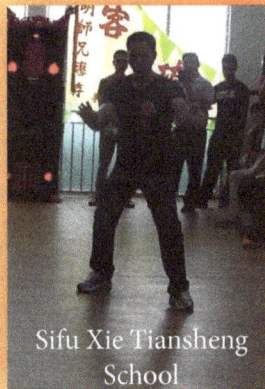

Sifu Xie Tiansheng School

HUIZHOU, GUANGDONG, CHINA

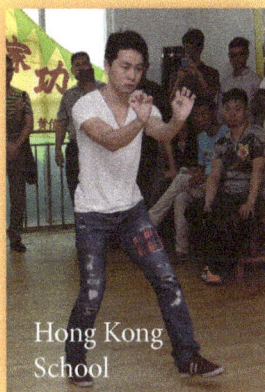

Hong Kong School

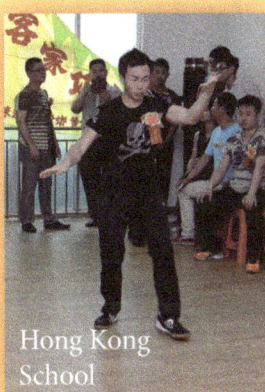

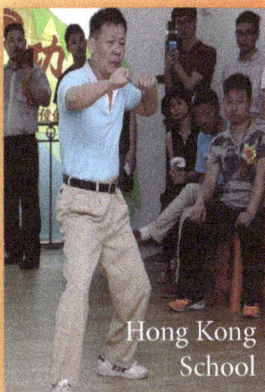

Hong Kong School

Hong Kong School

劉水功夫遺產在中國

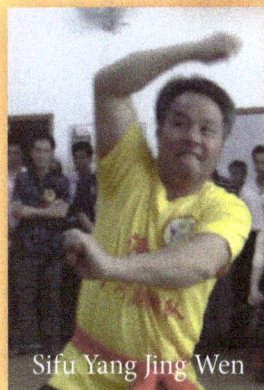

Sifu Yang Jing Wen

RDH

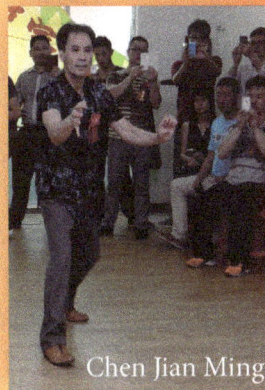

Chen Jian Ming

APOLOGIES TO THE MANY BROTHER-FRIENDS NOT
FEATURED HERE 此处没有都有兄弟的照片表示歉意

LOCAL HUIZHOU MEDIA INTRODUCED THE OPENING OF THE SCHOOL IN NEWSPAPER AND TV

當地報紙和電視臺推出新南派螳螂拳館

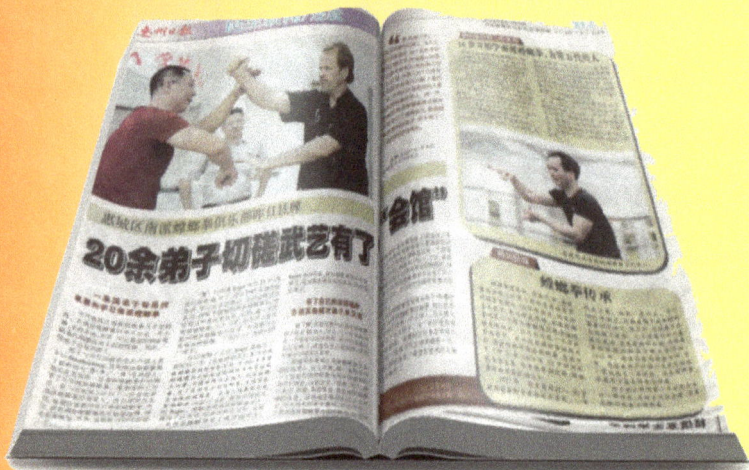

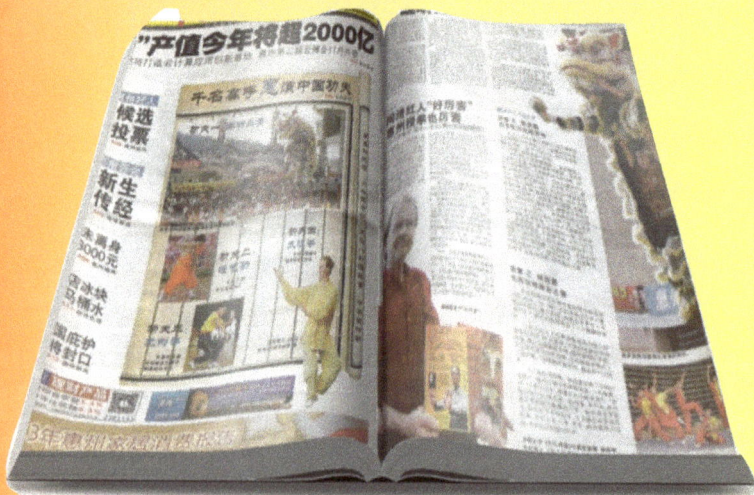

Huizhou Southern Mantis Boxing Association

惠州南派螳螂俱樂部

朱家螳螂派

陳建明
師傅

Sifu
Chen
Jianming

HAKKA MANTIS KUNGFU
CHU GAR, ZHU LIN TEMPLE

Roger D. Hagood
(美國人)
中文名稱
好厲害
師傅

江西竹林寺

電話:
15602628488

www.hakka-mantis.com

電話:
15986599499

陳建明師父和RDH師父的電話 – 如有意鍛煉請致電。

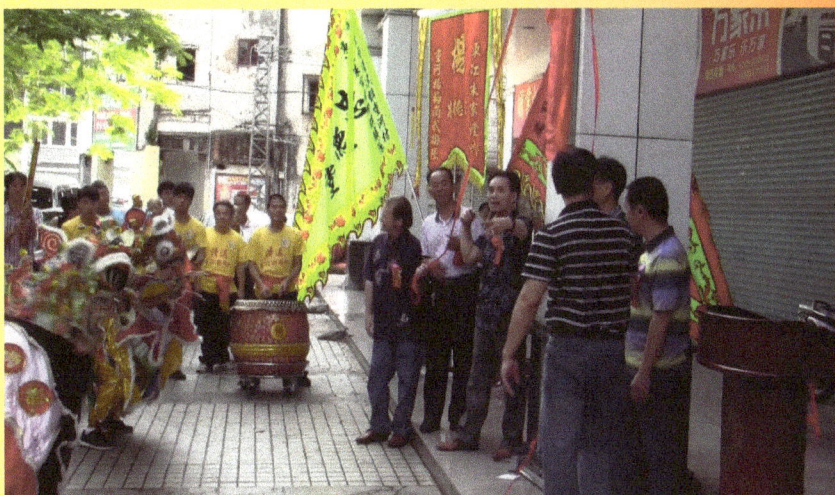

以上：揭開紅紙，打開樓下的廣告牌，陳健明，RDH和馬九華向楊維師父的麒麟回敬禮，當地官員在看著。

在選擇一個地點，並準備新的學校後，根據當地的風水先生選定的吉祥的日子和時間開幕。除了不計其數的本地嘉賓和知名人士，有大約15人來自楊維師父的麒麟藝術團專程從遙遠東莞市過來，及一組十五人左右，是李天來師父周家團隊，長途跋涉來自香港。所有的客人都在當地的方便的連鎖酒店過夜。這連鎖酒店幾乎出現在中國的每一塊土地上，每一條街道上。其中有一間連鎖酒店離開學校只有一排屋的距離，這對當地客人的或國際客人想拜訪惠州南螳螂拳協會和研究劉水的功夫遺產在中國的，提供方便的住宿。

揭幕儀式在上午9點及時開始，揭開覆蓋樓下戶外標誌的紅布，然後麒麟向標誌敬禮三次。麒麟表演後，其次是演講和儀禮。接著麒麟上學校的第四樓。麒麟再次敬禮，並揭開覆蓋門標誌的紅布。麒麟舞了一會兒，過後就直接去神台，再三敬禮並繼續表演一會兒，揭開了覆蓋神台的紅紙

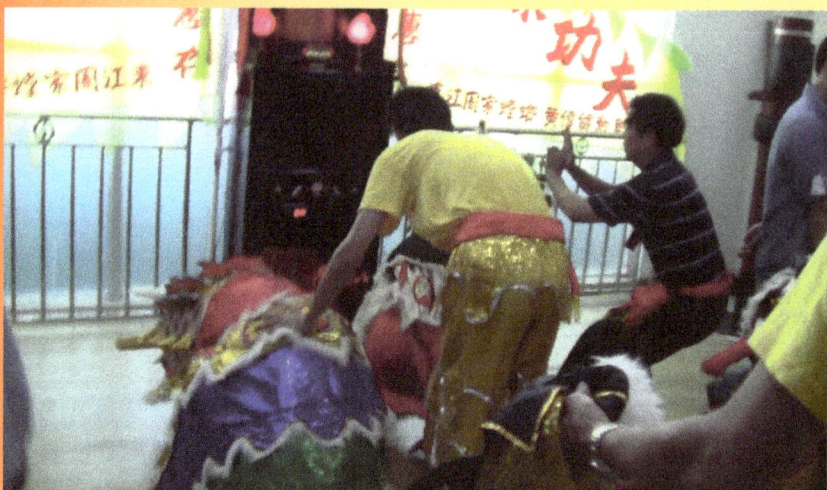

以上：Yang Wei師父的朱家麒麟在陳建明師父新開張的惠州南螳螂拳擊協會的神台敬禮。

這個紅色的揭幕是一種為學校帶來好運氣和吉祥的方法，因為紅標誌著生命的血液，在當地文化中象徵著好運氣。

打開新的學校的儀式及手續完成後，每個派別都先後的展示他們的技能。不僅新的朱家學校的學生表演，Yang Wei師父的朱家，和李天來周家都先後上來顯露幾手。此外，當地的師父和其他家的學生也表演他們的武藝風格。按照一般的規定，在其他人都表演後，身為主人的師父將表演。　所以我RDH，和陳建明師父輪流展示南螳螂拳法。我展示南螳螂混合式，陳師父展示朱家出第二式，Som Gin Yu Kiu。

有一位師父是 Chu Junsan 師父。　Chu Junsan 師父在場有個很特出的表現。他是朱家創始人朱亞南所發展出來的其中一個源流，這源流是不包括劉水師父的。其實，朱師父朱亞南的親戚。

大約中午時分，當每個人都被這半天的時間磨累，節目結束，並且附近的一個奇特的餐廳有個豐盛的午餐宴會等候大家。各個源流的人們都前去午餐宴會，並期待著另一個良辰吉日，再到惠州回訪南方螳螂拳擊協會。

這天，對於朱家和劉水功夫遺產中國，是歷史性的一天。這天，我也很榮幸的接受到陳建明師父的邀請，而成為這裡其中的一部分。事實上，在寫這篇文章期間，我繼續每天早上為這新的學校開門。同時我也積極尋求新的學生來發揚傳統。如果你是仁慈，並對朱家和南方螳螂有濃厚的興趣，請到惠州學校來訓練。

我堅信在我走了後，陳健明師傅將繼續教學和推廣他的新學校。他自小就是一位真正的武師。他才是將在他們的家鄉發揚劉水功夫遺產的人。

這是我們的任務，也是所有朱家拳擊好兄弟的任務，為子孫後代保存，促進和建立這藝術。加入我們的任務。從閱讀與研究開始。閱讀我的南螳螂書。我還計劃新的朱家書籍，包括Yellow Ox Tongue Staff，一個由劉水師父教下，難得一見的長棍套路。

請查詢www.hakka-mantis.com 以及其他網頁以知更多消息和詳情。還有數以百計的新的照片，是我寫這篇文章是還沒接收到的。為了您的興趣，我將在不久後為您發布，可能會在網站上發布。

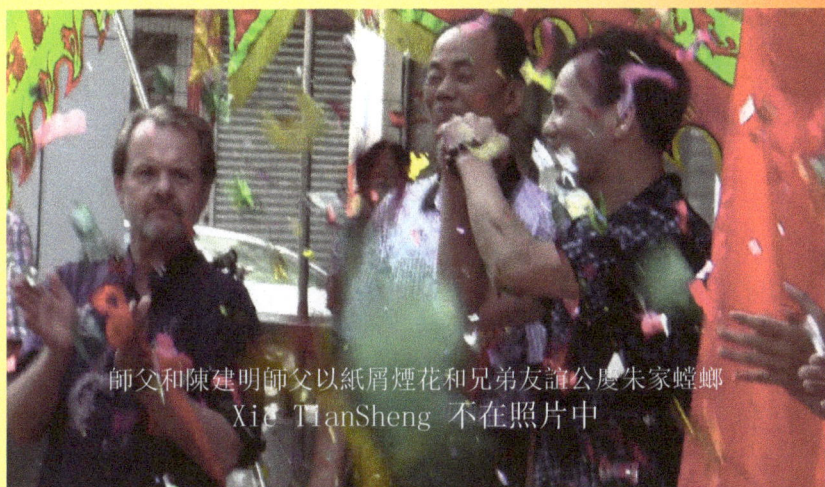

師父和陳建明師父以紙屑煙花和兄弟友誼公慶朱家螳螂
Xie TianSheng 不在照片中

請繼續閱讀關於朱家拳擊技術。

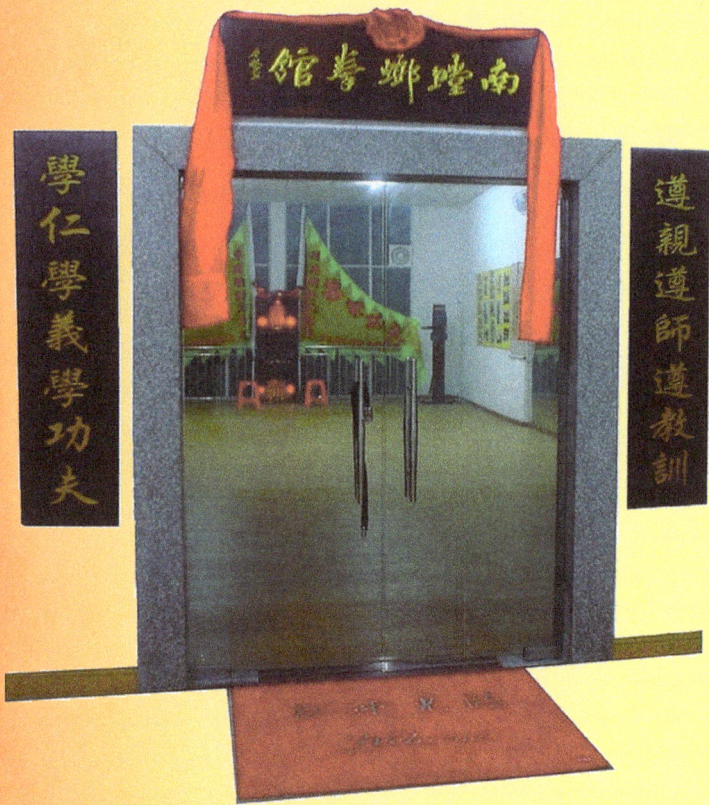

2013 Historic Chu Gar Event

The First Chu Gar 'Wuguan' Opens in Lao's Hometown

Some have described the opening of the first public Chu Gar School (wuguan) in Lao Sui's hometown as an historic event. And so it was for at least two reasons. Not the least was that I, the author of this book, RDH, a non-Chinese, was invited to cooperate in opening and teaching in the new Chu Gar School.

Secondly, this historic event brought together in cooperation three factions of Chu Gar: The Lao Sui Huizhou Clan of Chen Jian Ming, who opened the new School; the Yang Shou-Yang Wei Clan, and the Yip Sui 'Chow Gar' Clan of Li Tin Loi. All three factions participated in the opening of the first public Chu Gar School in Lao Sui's hometown. Well, four, because I, (RDH), am a Standing Chairman by appointment of Cheng Wan Sifu's Chu Gar Hong Kong Association.

40

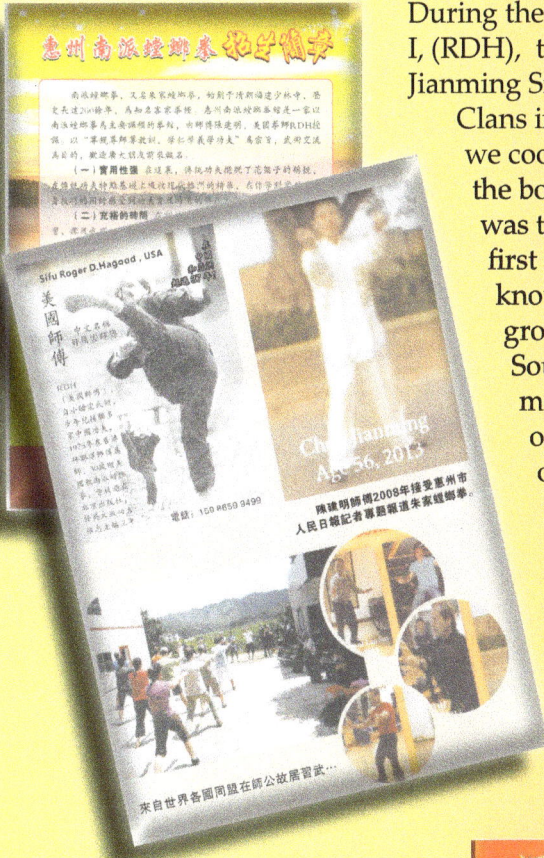

During the early months of 2013, I, (RDH), travelled to visit Chen Jianming Sifu and the Lao Sui Clans in their hometown and we cooperated to produce the book below. Chen Sifu was thinking to open the first Chu Gar Wuguan and knowing my strong background and interest in Southern Mantis invited me to cooperate in the opening and teaching of his School. A plan was hatched and an opening date and time was set according a local "Feng Shui" geomancer's auspicious signs! Read on to know more about this historic School.

Above: The School's opening promotional flyer featured Chen Jian Ming and RDH bios and detailed the School benefits and hours and a bit of Chu Gar history.

Right: The first book in the series of *Lao Sui's Martial Art Legacy in China* details Lao's family, history, the Chu Gar basic boxing and two forms. Future books will include the Yellow Ox Tongue Staff and Say Mun Ging Ging Four Gate Spring Power.

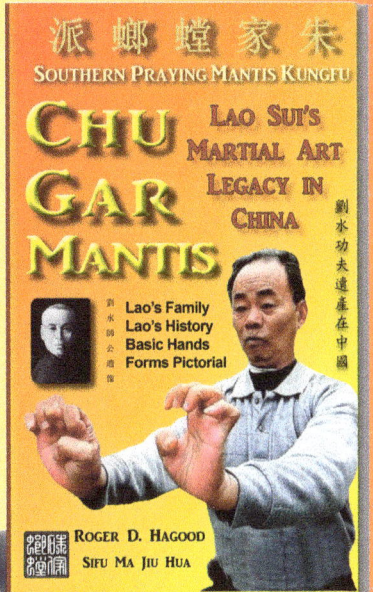

41

Two months of preparation went into the grand opening day of July first at 9 am. There was a great deal to be done in a short time. From ensuring legal compliance with all authorities, designing and creating a School from an empty building, to inviting guests and arranging their accommodations, two months is a relatively short time. Not to mention, that we travelled to call upon Yang Wei Sifu and requested his Unicorn troupe to perform the grand opening ceremonies.

Sidebar: Huizhou is ancient martial art city with records dating back to 800 AD and it is also the hometown of styles like Dragon and White Eyebrow. The old homesteads of both founders of these styles are still standing nearby the new Chu Gar School location. In addition, there are many Hakka stylists such as Li Gar, Li Gar Gao, Buddha Hand and others that practice locally today. Although, much of the old tradition has been replaced with Tae Kwon Do and even MMA.

陳建明師傅
惠州南派螳螂俱樂部

Yang Wei Sifu is a descendent from Yang Shou, one of Lao Sui's early students in Hong Kong. Yang Shou gained quite a reputation and even some have said that he, himself, may have been a third generation student of Chu Gar, from Wong Fook Go.

Today, near Guangzhou, the capital of Guangdong province, Yang Wei and the Yang Clan carry on in grand fashion the Hakka Chu Gar boxing tradition. They are also actively involved with Unicorn tradition and competitions.

So, Yang Wei, was invited to bring his troupe of some fifteen members and open the new Chu Gar School in Lao Sui's hometown. He was on top of the guest list which included many esteemed Sifu from the local Hakka groups, the local Huizhou Government's Wushu Association, and Hong Kong's Sifu Li Tin Loi from the Yip Sui "Chow Gar" clan.

Sifu Chen Jian Ming

Huizhou Southern Mantis Boxing School

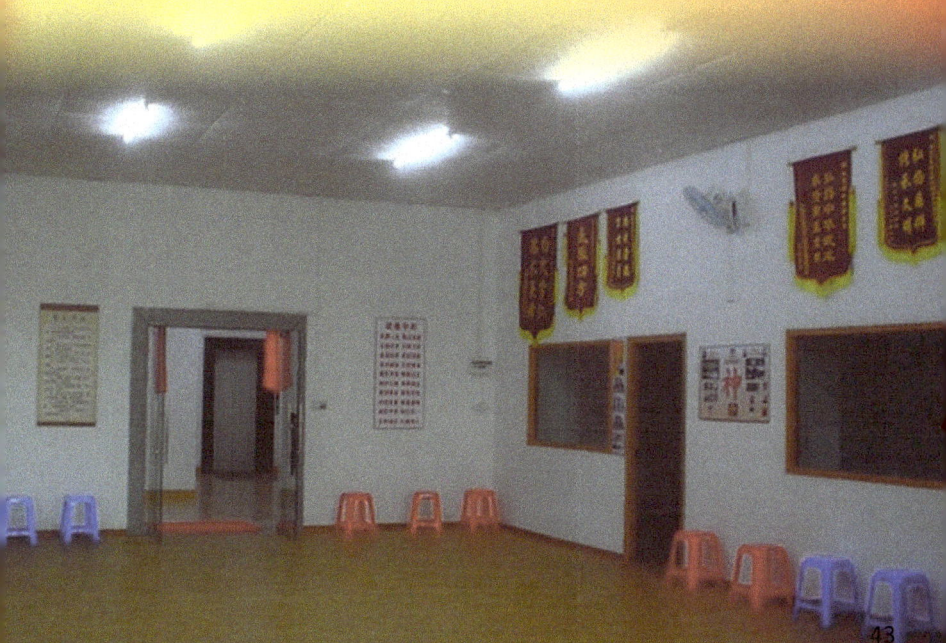

Above: The School's chart of history and lineage lists Lao Sui's legacy in both China and Hong Kong: Lao Sui 3rd generation, Ma Ming Sen 4th generation, Chen Jian Ming 5th generation, and RDH 6th generation among them. The photos show Lao Sui and Ma Ming Sen.

Below: Yang Wei Sifu's Chu Gar Unicorn Clan performs the grand opening and presents banners to Chen Jian Ming and RDH.

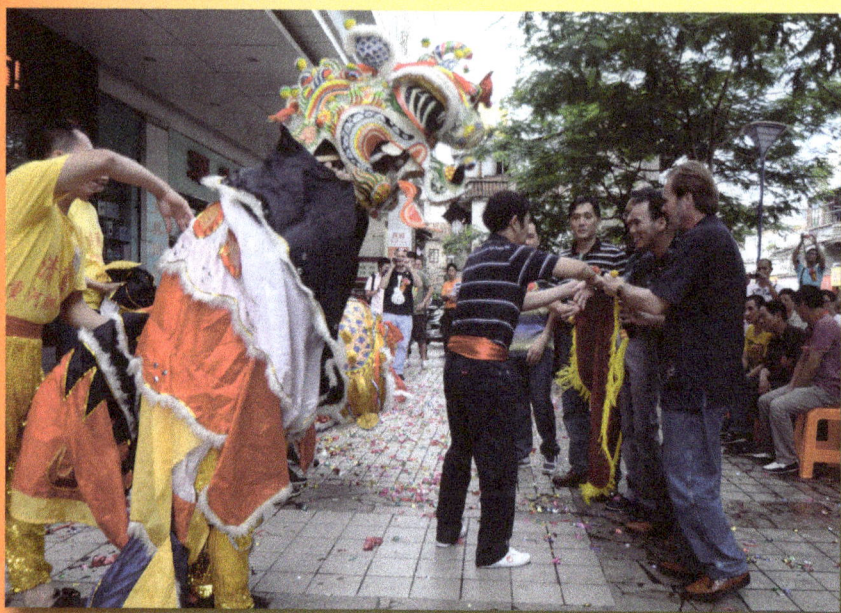

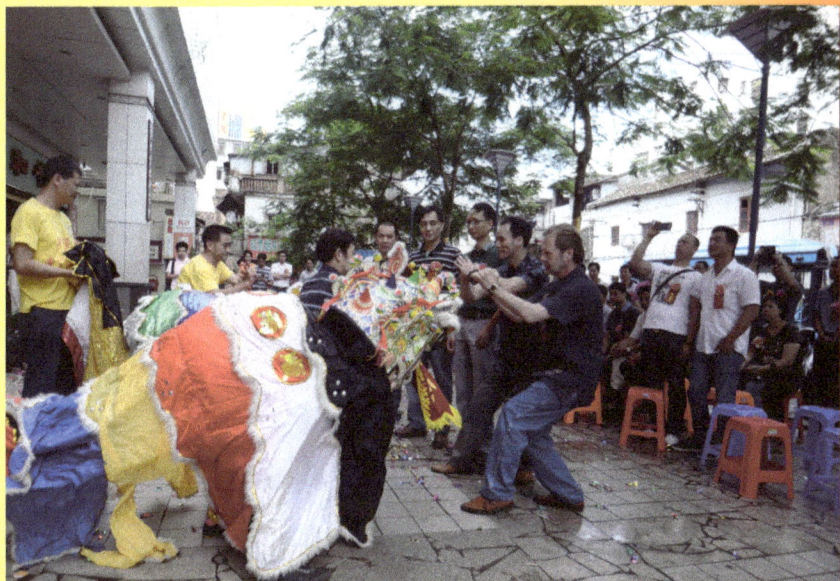

Above: Chen Jian Ming and RDH return salute to Yang Wei Sifu's Chu Gar Unicorn as local officials look on.

Below: The School Shrine states Chu Gar Mantis and Southern Praying Mantis Pai. The yellow standards were given by Li Tin Loi's Hong Kong "Chow Gar" faction. The history chart is shown on the left wall which includes Yip Sui and Li Sifu.

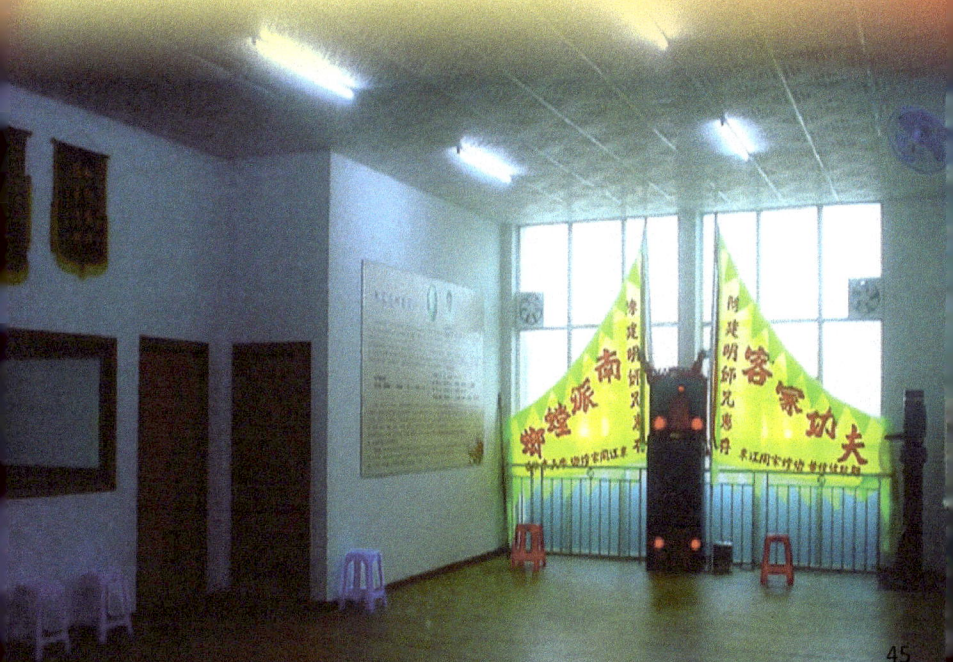

惠州南派螳螂俱樂部

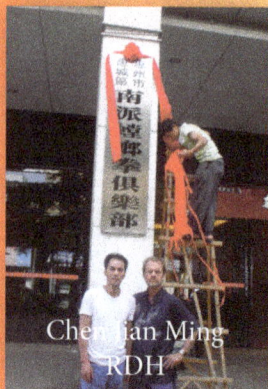

Chen Jian Ming RDH

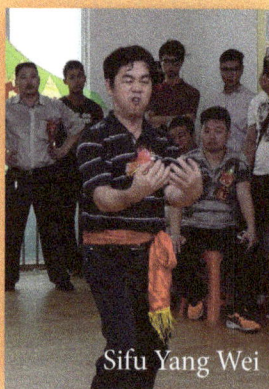

Sifu Yang Wei

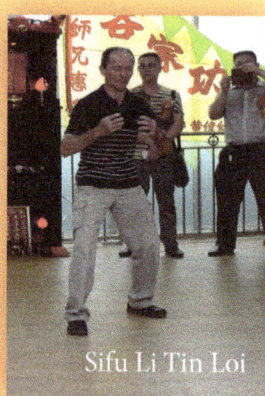

Sifu Li Tin Loi

GRAND OPENING JULY 1, 2013

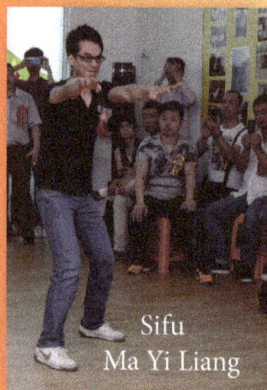

Sifu Ma Yi Liang

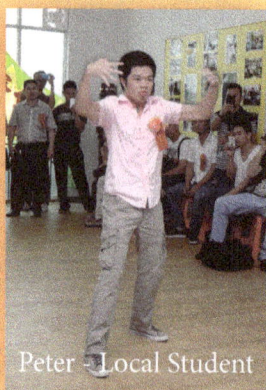

Peter - Local Student

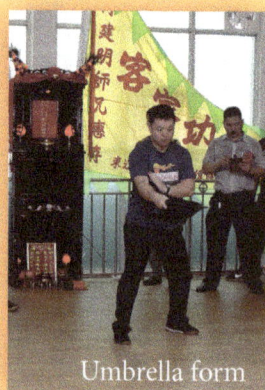

Umbrella form

LAO SUI'S CHU GAR MANTIS LEGACY IN CHINA

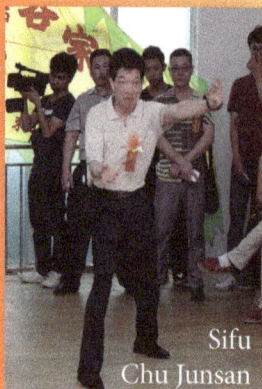

Sifu Chu Junsan

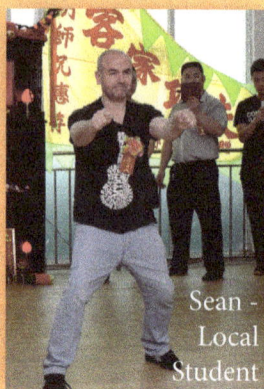

Sean - Local Student

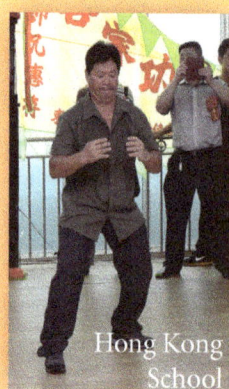

Hong Kong School

SIFU CHEN JIANMING'S CHU GAR SCHOOL IN HUICHENG

46

Huizhou Southern Mantis Boxing School

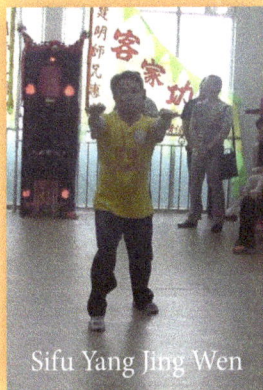

Sifu Yang Jing Wen

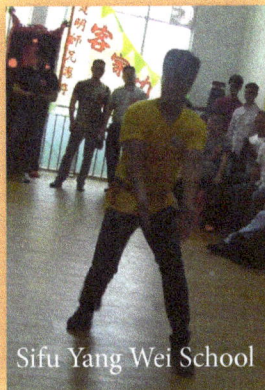

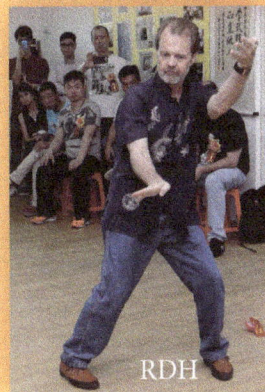

Sifu Yang Wei School

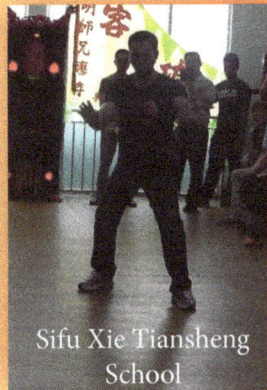

Sifu Xie Tiansheng School

Huizhou, Guangdong, China

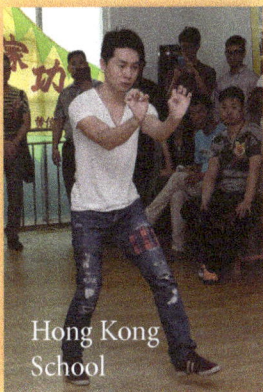

Hong Kong School

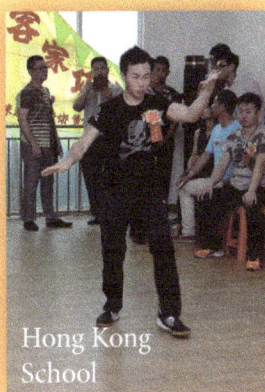

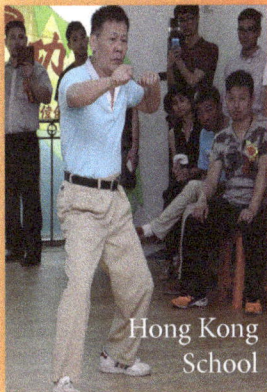

Hong Kong School

Hong Kong School

劉水功夫遺產在中國

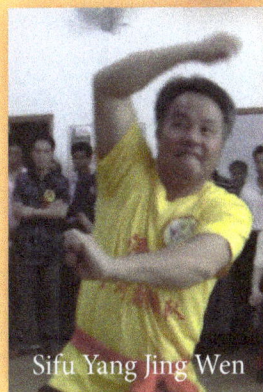

Sifu Yang Jing Wen

RDH

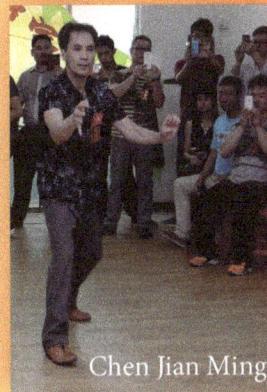

Chen Jian Ming

Apologies to the many brother-friends not featured here 此处没有都有兄弟的照片表示歉意

47

LOCAL HUIZHOU MEDIA INTRODUCED THE OPENING OF THE SCHOOL IN NEWSPAPER AND TV

當地報紙和電視臺推出新南派螳螂拳館

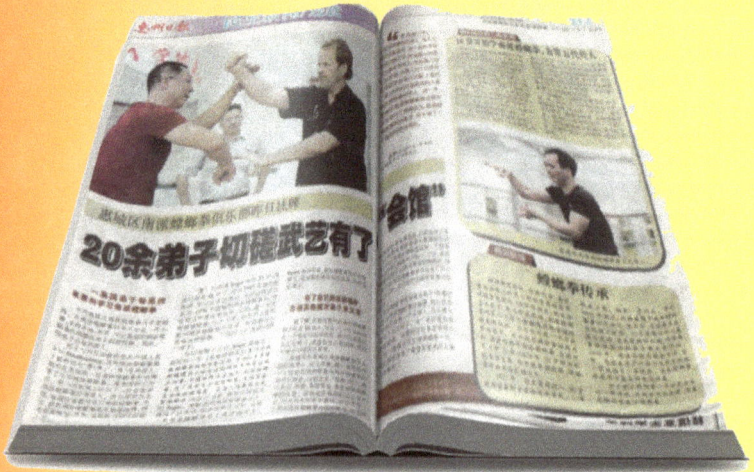

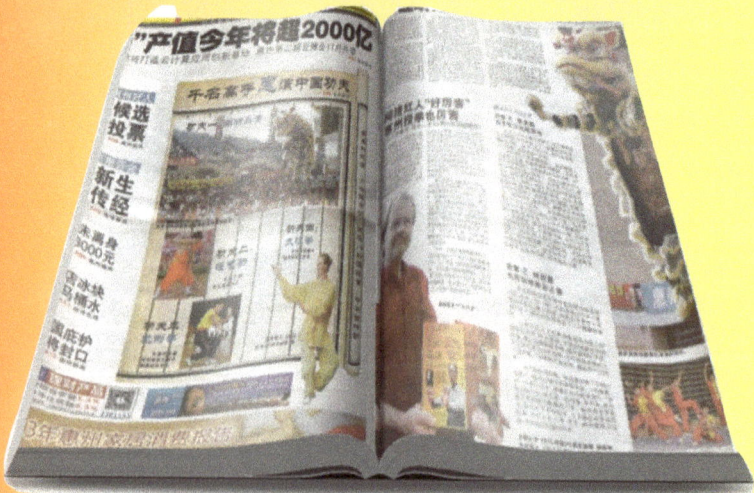

Huizhou Southern Mantis Boxing Association

惠州南派螳螂俱樂部

朱家螳螂派

陈建明
師傅
Sifu Chen Jianming

HAKKA MANTIS KUNGFU
CHU GAR, ZHU LIN TEMPLE

Roger D. Hagood
(美國人)
中文名稱
好属害
師傅

江西竹林寺

電話：
15602628488

www.hakka-mantis.com

電話：
15986599499

Chen Jian Ming And RDH Sifus' Numbers - call if you want to train!

48

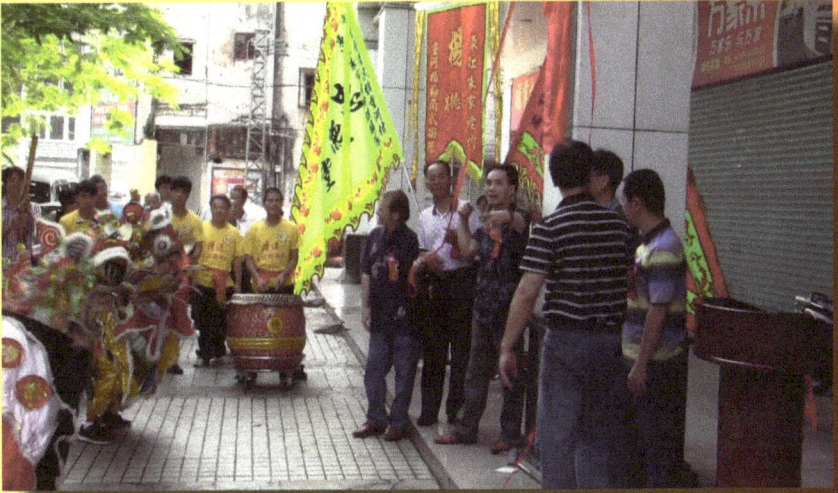

Above: Opening the downstairs billboard by removing the red, Chen Jian Ming, RDH and Ma Jihua return salute to Yang Wei Sifu's Chu Gar Unicorn as local officials look on.

After choosing a location and preparing the new School, it opened on an auspicious day and time as prescribed by a local geomancer. In addition to the multitude of local guests and dignitaries, there were some fifteen people in the Yang Wei Unicorn Troupe who travelled from distant Dongguan City and another fifteen or so in the Li Tin Loi 'Chow Gar' group from Hong Kong, who made the trek. All the guests stayed over night at a local Days Inn, a dandy and convenient chain hotel that has just about one on every block in all of China! One of these hotels is just one block from the School and very convenient for local or international guests who want to visit the Huizhou Southern Mantis Boxing Association and study Lao Sui's Legacy in China!

Ceremonies began promptly at 9 am with the unveiling of the red cloth covering the downstairs outdoor sign which then was saluted three times by the Unicorn. The dance was followed by speeches and formalities in accord with such a new establishment being opened, before the Unicorn proceeded up to the fourth floor double doors of the School. There, another Unicorn salute was made as the door signs covered in red were unveiled. With some fan fare and dance the Unicorn then proceeded straight to the Sun Toi or School Shrine where the same three salutes were performed while the Shrine

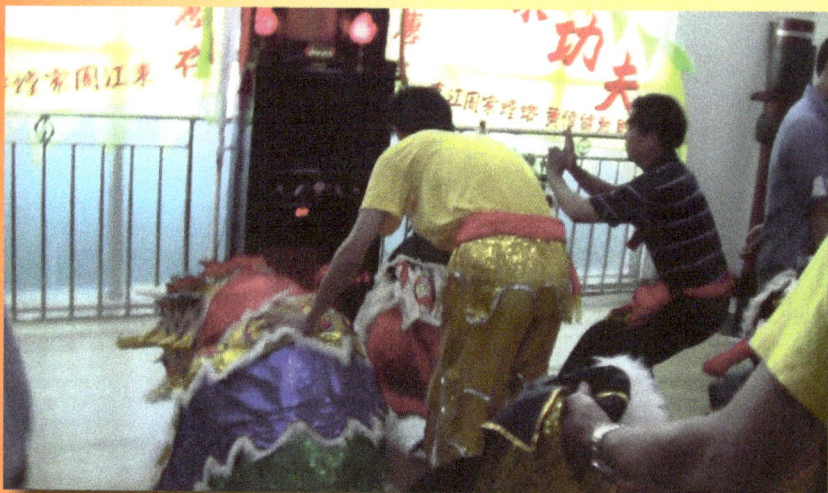

Above: Yang Wei Sifu's Chu Gar Unicorn salutes the Shrine during the opening of the Huizhou Southern Mantis Boxing Association of Chen Jian Ming Sifu.

covered in red paper was unveiled. All this red unveiling is a way of bringing good fortune and austerity to the new School, as red signifies the life blood of the body and good luck in local culture.

After the formalities of opening the new School were completed, then each faction took a turn at demonstrating their skills. Not only were students of the new Chu Gar School present to demonstrate, but also the Yang Wei Chu Gar Clan and the Li Tin Loi 'Chow' faction and each took their turn on the floor showing their hands. In addition, the local Sifu and students of other styles demonstrated their styles as well. As is custom, after everyone else has taken their turn showing off, then the host Sifu makes a performance and so I, RDH, and Chen Jian Ming each took a turn showing Southern Praying Mantis. I played a mixture of Southern Mantis and Chen Sifu played the Chu Gar second form, Som Gin Yu Kiu.

One notable performance was by Sifu Chu Junsan. He is descended from a separate stream of Chu Gar's founder Chu Ya Nan, that does not include Lao Sui. In fact, Chu Sifu is a relative of the founder of Chu Gar.

When everyone was worn out from the half day affair which ended around noon, a sumptuous lunch banquet was awaiting at a nearby fancy restaurant. From there each Clan went their on way awaiting another auspicious occasion to make a return visit to the Huizhou Southern Mantis Boxing Association.

It was an historic day for Chu Gar and Lao Sui's legacy of martial art in China, of which I was privileged to be a part by invitation of Chen Jian Ming Sifu. In fact, as of this writing, I continue to open the new School every morning and I am actively seeking new students to carry forward the tradition. Come to train in the Huizhou School if you are benevolent and with a strong interest in Chu Gar and Southern Mantis!

Chen Jian Ming Sifu will continue teaching and promoting in his new School long after I have gone, I am confident. He is a genuine martial artist since his childhood and it is he who will carry forward Lao Sui's Chu Gar legacy in their hometown.

It is our task, the task of all good Chu boxing brothers, to preserve, promote and build up the art for future generations. Join us in the task. It begins with self-study. Read my Southern Mantis books and I also plan new books on Chu Gar, including the Yellow Ox Tongue Staff, a rare pole form taught by Lao Sui.

Check the www.hakka-mantis.com and other websites for news and more information. There were many hundreds of photos of the new School opening that are not available to me as I write this. I will publish them for your interest soon, likely on the websites.

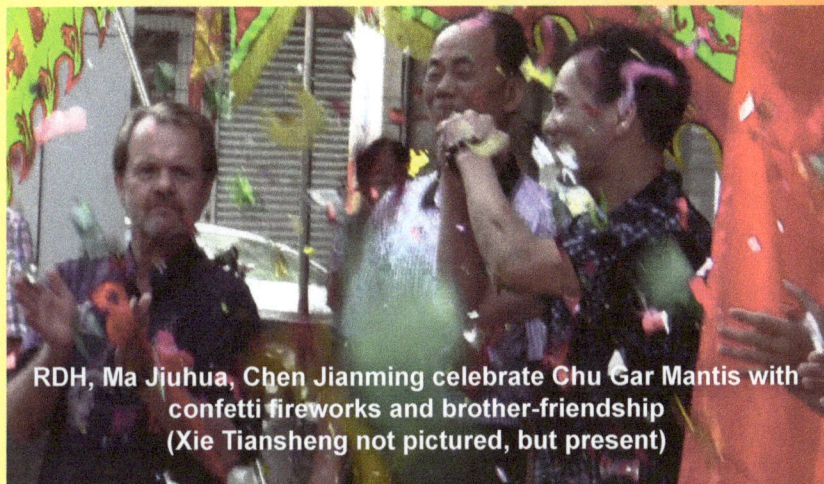

RDH, Ma Jiuhua, Chen Jianming celebrate Chu Gar Mantis with confetti fireworks and brother-friendship
(Xie Tiansheng not pictured, but present)

Read on now about the skills of Chu Gar boxing.

陈建明師傅

CHU GAR
SHORT DUMMY SET

In this chapter, gain a broad understanding of using the wooden man, as a second choice, in training. Chen Sifu's short dummy form teaches you to use the "ji ben gong" basic hand skills of Chu Gar Mantis on a wooden man. Simply apply the 12 basic hands in succession as shown - there is nothing mysterious, in this training. Just apply the hands center, left and right in sequence when you do not have a live partner.

Sifu Chen Jian Ming - Huizhou Chu Gar Mantis

About Wooden Man Dummy

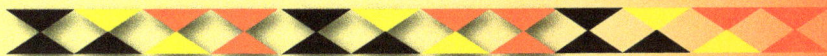

UNLIMITED CREATIVITY IN TRAINING APPARATUS

USA
Patent
5,665,035

SECRETS OF KUNG FU

AN OPPONENT WHO HIT
BRUCE LEE
IN THE TEMPLE

JACKIE CHAN
SHAOLIN WOODEN MEN

Wrestler Spars With Dummy

Fitted with springs and braces, this wooden sparring partner often plays, if resistance to the powerful holds of Everett Marshall of Detroit, Mich., heavyweight wrestler.

A WRESTLER in Detroit, Mich., prepares for bouts by practicing his holds on a wooden sparring partner. "Sandowstein," as the wooden dummy is called, is equipped with springs and braces that furnish resistant tension for the strong arms and legs of the wrestler, Everett Marshall.

54

ABOUT WOODEN MAN DUMMY

Live vs. Dead Power

As many types of training "dummies" and apparatus exist, as there are people who use them. Everyone has their own creative idea on what kind of device can be used to enhance their skills. And like the late Grandmaster Lam Sang said when asked which of his Southern Mantis students was right; there is no wrong - they are all right.

Any apparatus is a substitute for a "live dummy" - a live training partner. An apparatus, of any type, will always be a second-best ancillary aid. It takes the intellect, cunning, and the unpredictable reaction of a live person to refine superior skills in combat. Particularly, in Southern Praying Mantis, a 'live' training partner is necessary to refine the root, feeling hand (borrowing force), and the practice of striking the vital target points. Even the best made dummy with strong spring arms cannot react with human cunning.

Likewise, the "live wooden man" placed on slats for some springiness when hit, or the older, in the ground dummy, tamped loosely with rocks to have some slight movement when hit are still dead force. They cannot have the involuntary reaction of a real person nor can they learn or transmit feeling hand, borrowing force, or neutralizing - leading the opponent into emptiness.

Having said that, dummy and apparatus training can play an important part, since it is estimated that 80% of martial artists train solo, without a partner.

DUMMY HISTORY

Shaolin Tales

Everyone has read the history of 108 wooden men in the Shaolin Graduation Hall. Each of the 108 wooden men tested a different technique that was used by the monks. Later, after the Temple was burned and only five monks remained, Nun Ng Mui, one of the survivors, applied the 108 techniques to only one dummy and then taught her student Yim Wing Chun. Today's Wing Chun wall mounted dummy is said to be from a student of Yip Man because they didn't find it convenient to stick the dummy four feet into the ground while living in an apartment.

DUMMY HISTORY

North Mantis

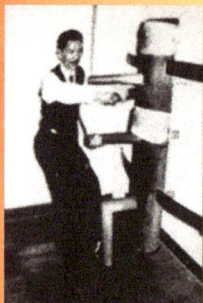

Northern Mantis players are known to use many kinds of apparatus. One notable, the late Master Chiu Chuk Kai (left circa 1960), of Taiji Mantis, in the 1940's, combined the Taizu Men and Taiji Praying Mantis techniques to create a Northern Mantis Wooden Dummy form that was inspired by his sworn brother's Wing Chun Kung Fu in Macau.

Master Chiu created a form that consists of 108 moves, which signifies cosmic balance in Chinese Buddhism, as well as, the historical connection to the Shaolin tradition. Chiu named the form "Shaolin Buddhist Wooden Dummy form" to commemorate his first masters, who were Buddhist monks in Shandong Province. It was solely Grandmaster Chiu's innovation to bring in the Wooden Dummy as a tool for his lineage. When training the dummy, he taught five plum blossoms: Mind must be bright, eyes must be clear, hands must be speedy, body must be committed, and footing must be precise.

Other Dummy Styles

Bruce Lee modified a Wing chun wooden dummy to include a modified neck and a metal leg. He was keen on using many and any kind of apparatus. Some say his use of an electrical apparatus to stimulate muscles might have factored into his death.

Many styles use dummies that cause action - reaction: balanced up, down, left, right, forward and back, weights, springs, sandbags, swinging arms, rotating 180 degree arms over, under, in and out, movable frames, spring loaded mechanisms, spinning arms, pulleys, etc. Any thing one can think of has probably already been done before.

Some say the traditional Wing Chun dummy should be made from oak with a length of 54", 9" diameter and weigh 110 lbs. The arms are 12" long with...etc, etc.

South Mantis

In Southern Mantis, dummies and apparatus do not have any requirements. Like using weapons, we say if the hand is skillful,

ABOUT WOODEN MAN DUMMY

anything you pickup will become a weapon. Most things can be your training apparatus with a little creativity and a lot of training.

There are some precedents. My Sifu, Mark Gin Foon, Kwongsai Mantis, used a dummy, in his School, in the late 70s / 80s. However, he did not teach a "dummy set". Students were free to play basic skills with the dummy, although, few did. His dummy was metal with springs, padded and covered in duct tape.

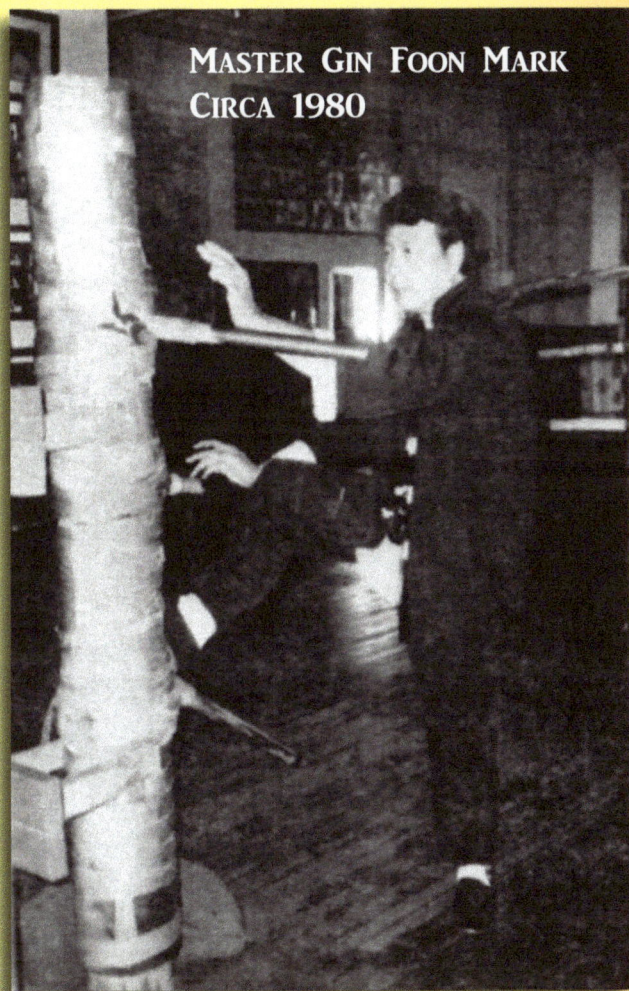

MASTER GIN FOON MARK
CIRCA 1980

My Kwongsai Mantis Sifu and Mark Foon Sifu's brother, Louie Jack Man, in the late 1970s, taught a "108 set" on a wooden man which looked much like the standard Wing Chun dummy.

His dummy set was fancy, not fluffy, and it included go behinds, low monkey steps, ghost chair steps, four corners, leg deflections, kicks, sweeps, etc. In short, it was based on the 18 Buddha Hands and included various Kwongsai Mantis footwork patterns. His later students also played the "108 Dummy Set" as shadowboxing, without the aid of the wooden man.

DUMMY HISTORY

South Mantis

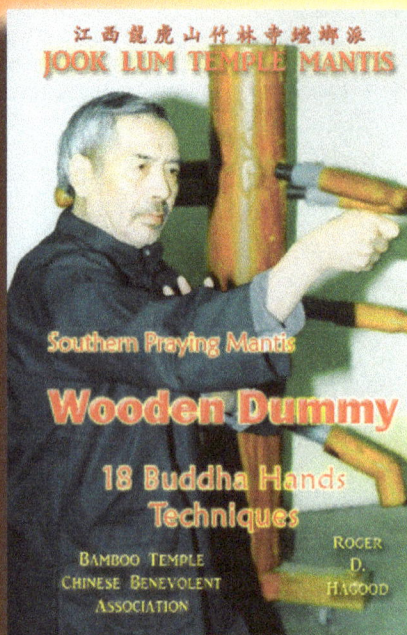

An upcoming Southern Mantis Press publication - Sifu Louie Jack Man

I once asked him, circa 1982, why he didn't just teach them the 108 two man set or at least just the 108 single man shadowboxing. His reply was he didn't want them to know that then - at that time. It was harsh, but that is what he said. He was old fashioned, in that way.

Today, 2014, the "Guang Wu Tang", Kwongsai Mantis Martial Hall of Wong Yu Hua Sifu, in Pingshan, China, has an almost standard wooden dummy wrapped in padding. It is not uncommon to find any kind of apparatus in a Mantis School, which may include, iron rings for the forearms, beans and rocks for finger training, large stones for finger grips, bamboo rollers for arm conditioning, iron bars for the arms to develop spring power ging, and more - limited only by creative ideas and materials.

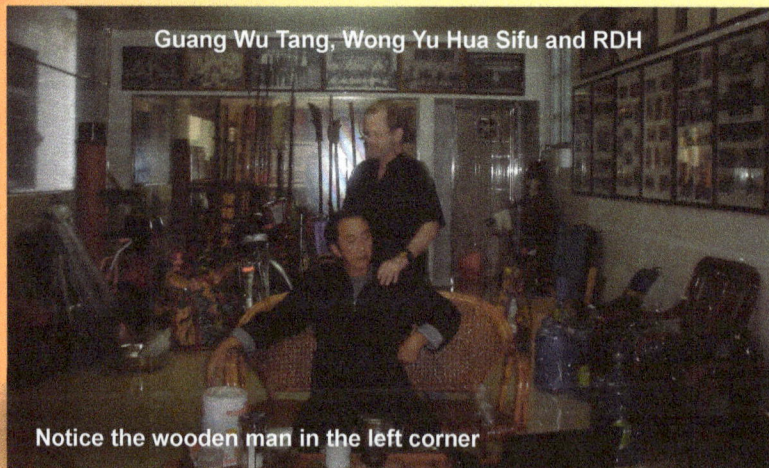

Guang Wu Tang, Wong Yu Hua Sifu and RDH

Notice the wooden man in the left corner

ABOUT WOODEN MAN DUMMY

Chu Gar Hakka Mantis

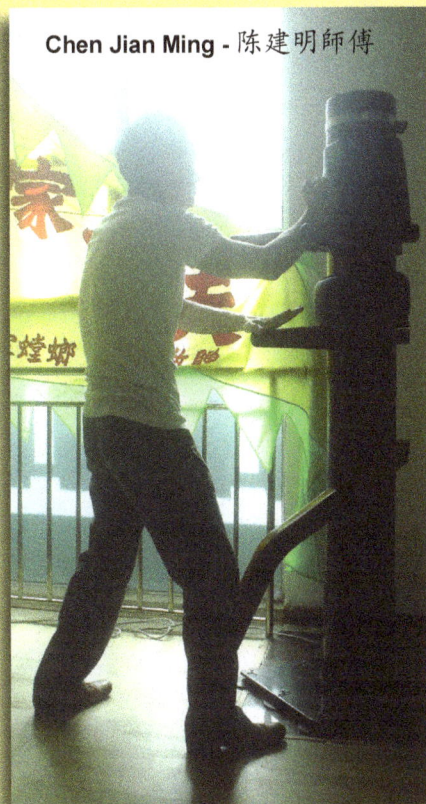
Chen Jian Ming - 陈建明師傅

Chen Jian Ming Sifu's Chu Gar Mantis Wuguan has a standard Wing Chun Dummy, too. His innovation has brought this Chu Gar "basic dummy hand" set to you. It is possible he will release a "long form dummy set" of Chu Gar Mantis in the future. And a DVD.

In this book, he details how to use the "ji ben gong" basic hand skills of Chu Gar Mantis, on a wooden man, and then he demonstrates, with Xie Tian Sheng Sifu, the applications of the dummy skills.

Like those before and likely after him, Chen Jianming's innovation will allow another generation to enjoy the benefits and training of Southern Praying Mantis.

History Conclusion

You may argue over the origin, history, size, weight, height, et al, of a wooden man, but in the end it is poppycock. 'Live' people come in all sizes and shapes and you should find a school with a variety of folks of all shapes, sizes, and colors with whom you can train hand to hand, regularly, daily if possible. This will give you a real advantage when you leave the wuguan, to the street.

Southern Mantis boxing is concerned with what is functional. If you do not have a training partner, then a broom stick stuck in a door jam may be useful. Play Sombogin (three steps forward): Start where you are, use what you have, do what you can. Get or make some kind of training apparatus, if you don't have a live training partner. Buy or make yourself a wooden man and train Chen Sifu's basic Chu Gar Mantis dummy hand set taught in this book. 59

DUMMY FUNCTION

Southern Mantis uses three bridges: crushing - force against force; borrowing force - feeling hand to use the opponent's strength against him; and evasive bridge - to neutralize or avoid.

One may play the wooden man using any or all three bridges and the four powers of float, sink, swallow, and spit. These principles are particularly important for people who must fend off a larger or stronger opponent or who simply wish to employ a more efficient and fluid method of defense, rather than using force against force. Study my book, "Eighteen Buddha Hands" for these principles and fundamental skills.

Crushing bridge, force against force, is a useful skill, so long as the opponent has less strength and skill than you. One simply may drive through, crush the opponent with any type of strike, regardless of his attack. One should take care not to develop "buffalo strength" when using crushing bridge, as short angles and deflections may still be employed when using this skill. Crushing bridge, refined, does not lead to brute strength wrestling, but is a way to swallow and spit the opponent's power simultaneously. It simply cheats his power while simultaneously driving straight through him. An example of crushing bridge is the "big gow choy" or "big hammer fist". It starts at the opponents head and simply drops like a sledgehammer down and through any defense.

When using the dummy to instill the ability to borrow the opponent's force and use it against him, that is to deflect or release an opponent's force against him, one must consider rooting, short hooking angles and deflections of the first and second hand, target practice of the vital points, timing (being important more than speed), and correct power. Not every skill requires 100% strength and exertion. Some skills were designed for turning force with less power. However, one should not think turning or borrowing force is magic. It takes power to turn power. Albeit, four ounces can turn one thousand pounds if the fulcrum and timing is right. With skilful feeling hand and borrowing force, one may control the opponent and strike him at will. This can be accomplished with a little idea and lot of training.

In borrowing force, one must be rooted in horse and posture. Without a root the hand will be deficient of power. Secondly, one

ABOUT WOODEN MAN DUMMY

must use the fulcrum of the second and first Mantis hands: the elbow and wrists, pulling power from the earth through the feet. Controlling the opponent's center is accomplished by controlling his elbows and knees. When this is skilful, one may need caution to keep from tearing the dummy from the wall or floor, without great exertion! It is simply a matter of intuiting the dummy's center point and applying pressure at the right leverage point to uproot. An example in Chu Gar is locking hands - one attaches hands and presses the opponent just enough so that when he resists he is easily uprooted or struck. One may learn to feel the correct angles when training over a protracted time with patience and a 'live' partner.

Using **evasive bridge** on the dummy requires multiple footwork patterns: Ghost chair side steps, 3 step, 4 corner, 8 direction, plum flower foot patterns, etc. Southern Mantis has many footwork patterns which may be employed beyond the basic steps. One simply neutralizes the opponent's attack with timing and steps by leading the opponent into an empty target. (See my Kwongsai Mantis Instructional DVD Volume Nine).

Additional Dummy training functions are :

- Toughness-conditioning of the forearms and limbs

- Visual reflexes - the eyes follow the hands; your eyes visually lock onto your opponent

- Contact reflexes - tactile sense with the dummy leads to feeling hand; contact leads to counter movement

- Execute blocks and strikes in concert, simultaneous with each other

- Correct footwork, distance, range, angle, deflection

HOW TO PLAY A DUMMY

Slowly at first without force to avoid injury. Gradually add force as the body is conditioned over time.

Remember the three bridges:

- Crushing - Force against force

HOW TO PLAY A DUMMY

- Borrowing - Deflection of the incoming force. Play the wooden man and avoid an opposing force head-on by hooks, angles, deflections, from larger to smaller and smaller

- Evading - Learn to move around the wooden man freely using footwork patterns and visualize timing to neutralize attacks

Gradually build your speed and power.

Learn to administer herbal treatment and massage therapy as needed to minimize injury from the wooden man. You are flesh.

Practice a warm up and cool down routine - start the wooden man slowly, if it is your warm up.

Minimum effort, maximum efficiency - learn economy of motion, do only what is necessary by negotiating the gates (sides) of the wooden dummy and striking at odd angles; if the opponent is weaker, then enter the center gate; if the opponent is stronger then enter from the side gates.

Think five petals of the plum flower:

- Mind keeps thinking

- Eyes keep observing

- Hands keep searching and seizing

- Body remains animated

- Feet keep evading

Be opportunistic and unpredictable remembering the six harmonies of external and internal work:

- Six Externals: Fists, eyes, arms, steps, body, strength

- Six Internals: Skill, tactics, boldness, swiftness, fierceness, practical

One should not forget and should endeavor to train the 18 Points of Internal Work, in each technique, when playing the dummy skills. Without having ingrained the principles, correct body posture, and fundamental hand skills, dummy work will not be useful or fruitful. If you know the Southern Mantis principles and fundamentals then

ABOUT WOODEN MAN DUMMY

almost any apparatus will become your dummy. Read my book "Eighteen Buddha Hands."

Understand and master each movement before moving to the next one. Step by step. Walk before you run the horse.

Keep in mind that Southern Mantis uses three bridges which you may train on the wooden man. First bridge strengthens the limbs and matches strength by using the superior crushing bridge with slight angles and deflections. Second bridge is not designed to strengthen the limbs but to train you to gain from one superior position to another by taking up the most suitable position through footwork and using second hand to borrow force. Third bridge requires light body skill, agility, and footwork to simply not be where the opponent is striking - he always finds an empty target - you are no longer where he thought to strike, when he arrives.

In qigong, one refines the audible breath to inaudible. In Southern Mantis, the four word secret of float, sink, swallow, and spit is first visibly large and small, short and tall, before refined into one economy of motion that does not need exaggeration. Do what only is necessary. In playing the wooden man dummy, the trainee who makes the noisiest movements while executing the dummy skills does not make the best use of it. Silence is golden.

Use the shoulder, hip, and knee moving in unison to deliver whole body power at once. Shake up the wooden man, your opponent, with whole body power. Hand and foot together arrive intently on the target, at once, with whole body power.

After you have, by rote, the wooden dummy routine - sequence, then train it is a shadowboxing routine, without the aid.

METHODS OF DUMMY TRAINING

Three Methods:

- Train on the dummy to develop the basic skills, proper form, use of footwork, eye hand coordination, etc.

- Practice the applications with a live partner in order to learn rooting, feeling hand, and target practice.

- Practice the dummy set beating the air as a form,

METHODS OF DUMMY SET TRAINING

as shadowboxing, solo training.

This is broken down into three categories:

- Hard (Crushing) Bridge- Blatant Attacks

- Soft (Borrowing Force) Bridge - confrontation and counter attacks

- Evasive (Neutralizing) Bridge and maneuvers

DUMMY BENEFIT

Techniques that are considered dangerous, even lethal, can be practiced without the fear of maiming your partner. You may train, as if facing a "real" opponent. Secondly, the wooden dummy has patience for you to repeat as necessary.

DUMMY TRAINING GOAL

Use the dummy, in absence of a real person, to refine the horse, posture and fundamental skills which you can then use when you have a live partner. This kind of dummy work will help you to move from the conscious to the instinctive level of training. Read the "Eighteen Buddha Hands" book to understand intuitive training.

PREREQUISITES

Before reading this book you should at least have studied:

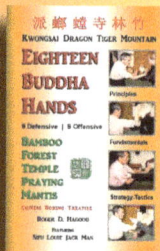

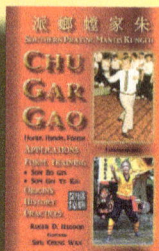

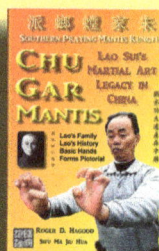

Amazon, Barnes and Noble, Books-A-Million

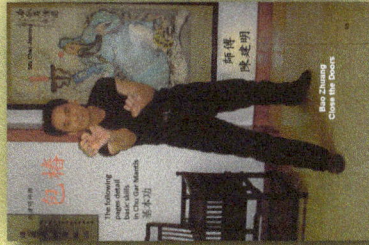

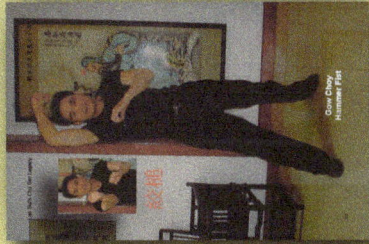

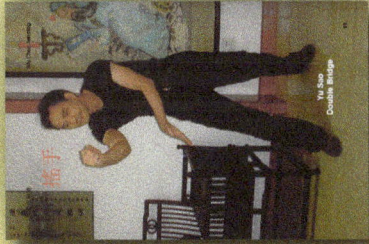

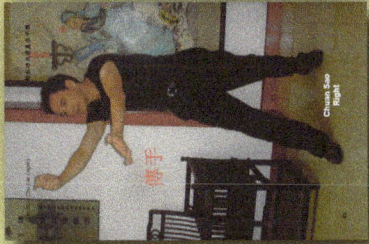

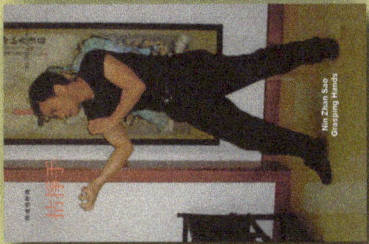

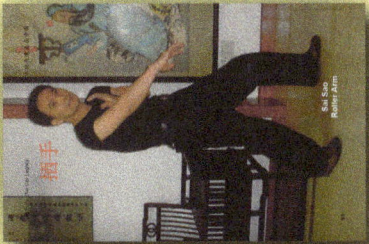

Play these basic hands in the L-R sequence shown, center, left, right of your dummy. Experiment. Find a live partner.

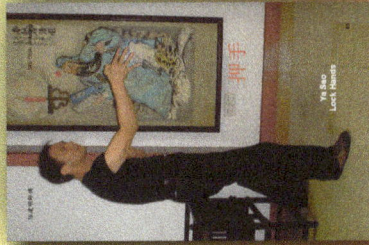

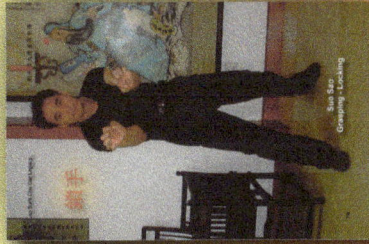

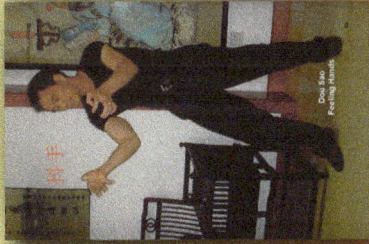

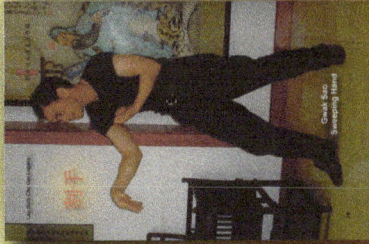

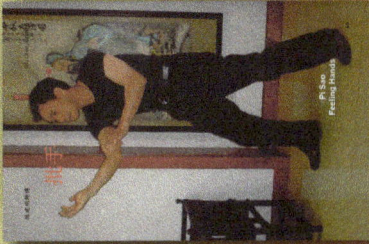

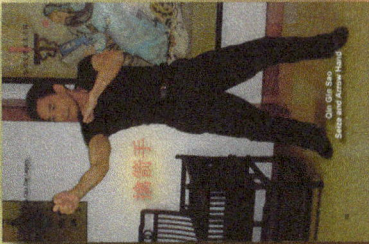

Sut Sau / Roller Arm

Cut Gar Sau / Sets and Arrow Hand

Nin Zhan Sao / Grasping Hands

Pi Sao / Feeling Hands

Chuen Sao / Right

Gwai Sao / Sweeping Hand

Yu Sao / Double Bridge

Dou Sao / Feeling Hands

Gau Choy / Hammer Fist

Sut Sao / Grasping & Locking

Bao Zhuang / Close the Doors

Ya Sao / Lock Hands

陈建明

UNLIMITED CREATIVITY IN TRAINING APPARATUS

USA
Patent
5,665,035

SECRETS OF KUNG-FU

AN OPPONENT WHO HIT
BRUCE LEE
IN THE TEMPLE

JACKIE CHAN
SHAOLIN WOODEN MEN

Wrestler Spars With Dummy

A WRESTLER in Detroit, Mich., prepares for bouts by practicing his holds on a wooden sparring partner. "Sandowstein," as the wooden dummy is called, is equipped with springs and braces that furnish resistant tension for the strong arms and legs of the wrestler, Everett Marshall.

Fitted with strong metal springs and braces, this wooden sparring partner, above, offers resistance to the powerful holds of Everett Marshall, a Detroit, Mich., heavyweight wrestler.

ABOUT WOODEN MAN DUMMY
关于木人桩

Live vs. Dead Power
生与死的能量

As many types of training "dummies" and apparatus exist, as there are people who use them. Everyone has their own creative idea on what kind of device can be used to enhance their skills. And like the late Grandmaster Lam Sang said when asked which of his Southern Mantis students was right; there is no wrong - they are all right.

许多人用许多不同类型的 "木人桩"和设备来培训。每个人都有自己的独到的方法来使用这些设备来使自己进步。 而正像林生师傅所说， 当他被问到他的哪个南螳螂弟子的使用方法是正确的时候， 他说没有谁是错的- 他们全都是对的。

Any apparatus is a substitute for a "live dummy" - a live training partner. An apparatus of any type will always be a second best ancillary aid. It takes the intellect, cunning, and the unpredictable reaction of a live person to refine superior skills in combat. Particularly in Southern Praying Mantis a 'live' training partner is necessary to refine the root, feeling hand (borrowing force), and the practice of striking the vital target points. Even the best made dummy with strong spring arms cannot react with human cunning.

在训练时， 任何设备都可以替代真人，但是设备毕竟不能达到真人训练的那种效果。 真人有智慧，计谋，和不可预知的反应，这些对于提高练武的水平都是很有利的。 尤其是在南螳螂拳派， 真人训练可以使步伐稳健， 身手矫捷， 锻炼人击中要害。 即便是最好的木人桩也不能与真人训练的效果相提并论。

Likewise, the "live wooden man" placed on slats for some springiness when hit, or the older, in the ground dummy, tamped loosely with rocks to have some slight movement when hit are still dead force. They cannot have the involuntary reaction of a real person nor can they learn or transmit absorbing energy, feeling hand, and borrowing force.

同样， 即使给木人桩附加弹性， 或者将旧的木人桩植入地里面， 周边用散石围住， 使木人桩在被打时可以移动, 这仍然是死能量。 这些木人桩不能有真人的预知反应也不能将能量转移或者是借力。

Having said that, dummy and apparatus training can play an important part, since it is estimated that 80% of martial artist train solo, without a partner.

话虽如此，木人桩和设备仍然是很重要的培训设备。据统计，80％的武术家平时都是靠自己独自训练的。

DUMMY HISTORY
木人桩的历史

Shaolin Tales
少林故事

Everyone has read the history of 108 wooden men in the Shaolin Graduation Hall. Each of the 108 wooden men tested a different technique that was used by the monks. Later after the Temple was burned and only five monks remained, Nun Ng Mui, one of the survivors, applied the 108 techniques to only one dummy and then taught her student Yim Wing Chun. Today's Wing Chun wall mounted dummy is said to be from a student of Yip Man because they didn't find it convenient to stick the dummy four feet into the ground while living in an apartment.

每个人有读那个108木人 在少林毕业馆的历史. 每个108木人考和尚用的不同技术. 少林寺被火烧之后，只留五个和尚，其中一个是吴梅尼姑. 吴梅尼姑运用108技术在一个木人桩. 过后教严咏春. 今天的咏春墙壁安装的桩说是叶问一名学生创的. 这因为是他们发觉不方便木人桩钻4尺入地当住在高楼大厦.

North Mantis
北螳螂派

Northern Mantis players are known to use many kinds of apparatus. One notable, the late Master Chiu Chuk Kai (left circa 1960), of Taiji Mantis, in the 1940's, combined the Taizu Men and Taiji Praying Mantis techniques to create a Northern Mantis Wooden Dummy form that was inspired by his sworn brother's Wing Chun Kung Fu in Macau.

北螳螂武术家是已知用许多不同设备. 一名太极螳螂师傅，赵竹溪宗师（左大约1960年），在1940时代，结合太祖门派和太极螳螂的技术, 创了北螳螂木人套拳，这套拳是他的结拜兄弟在澳门咏春派灵感的.

Master Chiu created a form that consists of 108 moves, which signifies cosmic balance in Chinese Buddhism as well as the historical connection to the Shaolin tradition. Chiu named the form "Shaolin Buddhist Wooden Dummy form" to commemorate his first masters, who were Buddhist monks in Shandong Province. It was solely Grandmaster Chiu's innovation to bring in the Wooden Dummy as a tool for his lineage. When training the dummy he taught five plum blossoms: Mind must be bright, eyes must be clear, hands must be speedy, body must be committed, and footing must be precise.

赵宗师创了一套拳有108技术，象征禅宗宇宙的平衡，以及历史上少林的关系．赵宗师指名那套拳 "少林禅宗木人桩"，纪念他的前辈大师，他们都是山东禅宗和尚．这是完全赵宗师革新来用木人桩作为他的门派设备．培训木人桩时，他教五梅花：心要光，眼要清，手要快，身要献，和步要准．

Other Dummy Styles
其他木人桩式

Bruce Lee modified a Wing chun wooden dummy to include a modified neck and a metal leg. He was keen on using many and any kind of apparatus. Some say his use of an electricity apparatus to stimulate muscles might have factored into his death.

李小龙修改了咏春木人桩，他加了改动的颈和铁腿．他敏锐用任何设备来培训．有人说，他使用的电力设备来刺激肌肉可能成因他的死亡．

Many styles often use dummies that cause action - reaction: balanced up, down, left, right, forward and back, weights, springs, sandbags, swinging arms, rotating 180 degree arms over, under, in and out, movable frames, spring loaded mechanisms, spinning arms, pulleys, etc. Any thing one can think of has probably already been done before.

许多功夫派用会有行动反应的木人桩：平衡上，下，左，右，前进和后退，重量，弹簧，沙包，摇臂，180度转臂以上，以下，以内，以外，可移动的桩，弹簧的机理，移动的臂，滑轮，等等．任何设备人能想到可能已经被试了．

Some say the traditional Wing Chun dummy should be made from oak with a length of 54", 9" diameter and weigh 110 lbs. The arms are 12" long with...etc, etc.

有人说，传统咏春木人桩应该是用橡木做的，是长度54寸，直径9寸及重量110英镑．手臂应该是12寸等等，等等．

South Mantis
南螳螂派

In Southern Mantis, dummies and apparatus do not have any requirements. Like using weapons, we say if the hand is skillful, anything you pickup will become a weapon. Anything can be your training apparatus with a little creativity and a lot of training.
在南螳螂派，木人桩和其他设备没有任何需求．像用任何武器，我们说如果手有熟劲，任何东西可以作武器．任何东西可以作设备只要用创造和训练．

However, there are some precedents. My Sifu, Mark Gin Foon, Kwongsai Mantis, used a dummy in his School in the late 70s / 80s. However, he did not teach a "dummy set". Students were free to play basic skills, although, few did. His dummy was metal with springs, padded and covered in duct tape. And my Kwongsai Mantis Sifu and Mark Foon Sifu's brother, Louie Jack Man, in the late 1970s, taught a "108 set" on a wooden man which looked much like the standard Wing Chun dummy.
但是在南螳螂派有前例．我的师傅，江西螳螂麥振宽，在70,80时代时,在他的武管有用木人桩．但是，他没有教套路．他的学生自由练基本功，虽然没有只个练．他的木人桩是铁做的，被胶带盖垫了．我的江西螳螂师傅,同时也是麥振宽的师弟，雷泽民在70时代末，教‘108套’用木人桩类似普通咏春木人桩．

Photo: Master Gin Foon Mark Circa 1980.
照片：麥振宽师傅大约1980．

His dummy set was fancy, not fluffy, and it included go behinds, low monkey steps, ghost chair steps, four corners, leg deflections, kicks, sweeps, etc. In short, it was based on the 18 Buddha Hands and included various Kwongsai Mantis footwork patterns. His later students also played the "108 Dummy Set" as shadowboxing, without the aid of the wooden man.
他的木人桩套路是花式的，但不是蓬松．这个套路有去桩的后面，低猴子步，鬼椅子步，四个角，腿打歪，踢，扫，等等．总之，是踞18佛手和许多江西螳螂脚步式．他的后学生也有练‘108套’空拳，没有用木人桩．

South Mantis
南螳螂派

Photo: An upcoming Southern Mantis Press publication - Sifu Louie Jack Man
照片：将来的南螳螂派出版社出版 -雷泽民师傅.
I once asked him, circa 1982, why he didn't just teach them the 108 two man set or at least just the 108 single man shadowboxing. His reply was he didn't want them to know that then - at that time. It was harsh but that is what he said. He was old fashioned in that way.
我有一次问他，大约1982年，他为什么不教他们108双人套路, 或者至少教108单人套路. 他回答说，在那个时候他不想让他们知道. 这是苛但是那是他所说的. 他是在那方面老时尚.

Today, 2013, the "Guang Wu Tang", Kwongsai Mantis Martial Hall of Wong Yu Hua Sifu in Pingshan, China, has an almost standard wooden dummy wrapped in padding. It is not uncommon to find any kind of apparatus in a Mantis School, which may include, iron rings for the forearms, beans and rocks for finger training, large stones for finger grips, bamboo rollers for arm conditioning, iron bars for the arms to develop spring power ging, etc.
今天，2013年，‘光武堂’，中国坪山黄耀华江西螳螂派师傅的武术堂，有一个几乎普通的木人桩被垫了. 在螳螂武术堂，有许多不同的设备，其中可能包括，铁环，豆和石头训练手指，大石头训练手指握力，竹卷训练手臂，铁棒训练手臂发劲，等等.

Photo: Guang Wu Tang, Wong Yu Hua Sifu and RDH, 2012, January. Notice the wooden man in the left corner.
照片：光武堂，黄耀华师傅和RDH，2012 一月. 注意木人桩在左角.

Chu Gar Hakka Mantis
朱家客家螳螂

Chen Jian Ming Sifu's Chu Gar Mantis Wuguan has a standard Wing Chun Dummy too. His innovation has brought this Chu Gar "basic dummy hand" book to you. It is possible he will release a "long form dummy set" of Chu Gar Mantis in the future.
在陈健明师傅的朱家螳螂物管也有一个咏春木人桩. 他的创新带来了这个朱家"基本木人桩手法. 有可能未来他会发布朱家螳螂的"木人桩长套路".

In this book, he details how to use the "ji ben gong" basic hand skills of Chu Gar Mantis on a wooden man and then he demonstrates with student, Sean Robinson, the applications of the dummy skills.
在这本书中，他详细用木人桩解释朱家螳螂"基本功" 基本手法.
然后他和学生,Sean Robinson, 示范手法的用法.

Like those before and likely after him, Chen Jianming's innovation will allow another generation to enjoy the benefits and training of Southern Praying Mantis.
像那些在他之前和之后，陈建明的创新将来让下一代享受南螳螂培训的好处.

History Conclusion
历史结论

You may argue over the origin, history, size, weight, height, etc of a wooden man, but in the end it is poppycock. 'Live' people come in all sizes and shapes and you should fi nd a school with a variety of folks of all shapes, sizes, and colors with whom you can train hand to hand, regularly, daily if possible. This will give you a real advantage when you leave the wuguan to the street.
你可能会议论木人桩的来源，历史，尺寸，重量，高度，等等，但也是胡说. 活人有各种尺寸，你应该找学校训练手法. 当在街上给你优越.

Southern Mantis boxing is concerned with what is functional. If you do not have a training partner, then a broom stick stuck in a door jam may be useful. Play Sombogin (three steps forward): Start where you are, use what you have, do what you can. Get or make some kind of training apparatus if you don't have a live training partner. Buy or make yourself a wooden man and train Chen Sifu's basic Chu Gar Mantis dummy hand set taught in this book.
南螳螂拳最重要的是能用. 如果你没有训练伴，可以用扫帚棍作训练培训. 三步前：开始在哪里，用什么你有，做什么你可. 如果没有训练伴，你可以做装置来训练. 做或买个木人桩，训练这本书的陈师傅朱家螳螂"基本功" 基本手法.

DUMMY FUNCTION
木人桩用法

Southern Mantis uses three bridges: crushing - force against force; borrowing force - feeling hand to use the opponent's strength against him; and evasive bridge - to neutralize or avoid.
南螳螂用三个桥：力对力；借力 – 摸手借对方的力来对付他；以吞桥 – 抵消或避开.

One may play the wooden man using any or all three bridges and the four powers of float, sink, swallow, and spit. These principles are particularly important for people who must fend off a larger or stronger opponent or who simply wish to employ a more efficient and fluid method of defense, rather than using force against force. Study my book, "Eighteen Buddha Hands" for these principles and fundamental skills.
谁练木人桩使用的任何或全三桥和力量（浮, 沉, 吞, 吐）. 这些原理是特别重要对人对付比较高大的对方或想用比较高效和流动的防手，而不想用力对力. 读我的书，'十八佛手'，学习原理和基本功夫.

Crushing bridge, force against force, is a useful skill, so long as the opponent has less strength than you. One simply may drive through, crush the opponent with any type of strike, regardless of his attack. One should take care not to develop "buffalo strength" when using crushing bridge as short angles and deflections may still be employed when using crushing bridge. Crushing bridge refined does not lead to brute strength wrestling but is a way to swallow and spit the opponent's power simultaneously. It simply cheats his power while simultaneously driving straight through him. An example of crushing bridge is the "big gow choy" or "big hammer fist". It starts at the opponents head and simply drops like a sledgehammer down and through his any defense.
用力对力是一个有效的技能，只要对方比较弱. 你可以用任何手法来对付他，不关他的攻击. 用力对力时，不要用牛力. 但用小角度和偏转. 力对力是一个方法同时来吞和吐对方的力量. 这只是用对方的力量同时来穿过他. 一个例子是大锤拳. 大锤拳于头开始落下似大锤，穿过任何防御.

When using the dummy to instil the ability to borrow the opponent's force and use it against him, that is to deflect or release an opponent's force against him, one must consider rooting, short hooking angles and deflections of the first and second hand, target practice of the vital points, timing being important more than speed, and correct power. Not every skill requires 100% strength and exertion. Some skills are designed for turning force with less power. However, one should not think turning or borrowing force is magic. It takes power to turn power. Albeit, four ounces can turn one thousand pounds if the fulcrum and timing is right. With skilful feeling hand and borrowing force, one may control the opponent and strike him at will. This can be accomplished with a little idea and lot of training.

用木人桩训练借对方的力量来针对他时，就是说偏转或者用对方的力量来针对他，你要考虑生根，小角度钩拳和偏转的第一和第二段螳螂手，打中目标关键点，计时比较重要过速度，和正确的力量．不是每一个手法需要用100％力量．有些手法借对方的力量所以用少力．但是借对方的力量并不是魔法但需要对方的力量．四两拨千斤如果支点和计时是准确．以熟练的摸手和借力，你可以容易的控制和打击对方．这可以完成通过很多训练．

In borrowing force, one must be rooted in horse and posture. Without a root the hand will be deficient of power. Secondly, one must use the fulcrum of the second and first Mantis hands: the elbow and wrists, pulling power from the earth through the feet. Controlling the opponent's center is accomplished by controlling his elbows and knees. When this is skilful, one may need caution to keep from tearing the dummy from the wall or floor, without great exertion! It is simply a matter of intuiting the dummy's center point and applying pressure at the right leverage point to uproot. An example in Chu Gar is locking hands - one attaches hands and presses the opponent just enough so that when he resists he is easily uprooted or struck. One may learn to feel the correct angles when training over a protracted time with patience and a 'live' partner.

如果要借力，你必要有生根 – 马步和姿势．如果没有生根，手就无力量．还有，你必要用第一和第二段螳螂手做支点：手肘和手腕，用脚吸收地的力．控制对方的手肘和手腕就可以控制他的中线．有这个技能，你需要小心打破坏木人桩．你需要知道木人桩的中线和施加压力来铲根．例子，朱家螳螂的锁手 – 你按促对方，当他抗拒他就容易铲根或者被打．你可以学习感觉到正确的角度但需要忍耐培训长时间和有'活'培训伴．

Using evasive bridge on the dummy requires multiple footwork patterns: Ghost chair side steps, 3 step, 4 corner, 8 direction, plum flower foot patterns, etc. Southern Mantis has many footwork patterns which may be employed beyond the basic steps. One

simply neutralizes the opponent's attack with timing and steps
by leading the opponent into an empty target. (See my Kwongsai
Mantis Instructional DVD Volume Nine).
在木人桩用逃避桥需要不同步法：侧步，三步，四角，八方向，梅花
脚步法等等. 南螳螂有很多步法，用法超出基本的脚步. 你用计时和
步法来抵消对方的攻击以带对方到空虚. （看我的江西螳螂教学DVD第
九卷）.

Additional Dummy training functions are :
• Toughness-conditioning of the forearms and limbs
• Visual refl exes - the eyes follow the hands; your eyes visually
lock onto your opponent
• Contact reflexes - tactile sense with the dummy leads to feeling
hand; contact leads to counter movement
• Execute blocks and strikes in concert, simultaneous with each
other
• Correct footwork, distance, range, angle, deflection
另外木人桩的训练作用：
• 　　硬化力 － 训练手臂和四肢.
• 　　视觉的反射性 －眼睛跟着手；眼睛锁定对方.
• 　　触摸的反射性 － 训练摸手；触摸跟着反应.
• 　　同时防手和攻击.
• 　　正确的马步，远方，范围，角度，偏转.

HOW TO PLAY A DUMMY
如何训练木人桩

Slowly at first without force to avoid injury. Gradually add force as
the body is conditioned over time.
先开始时，别用力以避免受伤. 慢慢如身体训练强硬在加力量.

Remember the three bridges:
• Crushing - Force against force
• Borrowing - Deflection of the incoming force. Play the wooden
man and avoid an opposing force head-on by hooks, angles,
deflections
• Evading - Learn to move around the wooden man freely using
footwork patterns and visualize timing to neutralize attacks.
三个桥：

- 破碎力 － 用力对力.
- 借力 － 偏转来的力量. 避免正面反力, 但用钩拳, 角度, 偏转.
- 逃避 － 学习用步法在木人桩四处移动. 想象用计时来抵消攻击.

Gradually build your speed and power.
慢慢加速度和力量.

Learn to administer herbal treatment and massage therapy as needed to minimize injury from the wooden man. You are flesh.
学会用中药和按摩如减低外伤.

Practice a warm up and cool down routine - start the wooden man slowly if it is your warm up.
练习热身和冷却例行 － 开始训练木人桩时, 练速度慢慢起来.

Minimum effort, maximum efficiency - learn economy of motion, do only what is necessary by negotiating the gates (sides) of the wooden dummy and striking at odd angles; if the opponent is weaker, then enter the center gate; if the opponent is stronger then enter from the side gates.
最小的功力, 最高的效率 － 学习经济动作, 只做有必要来通过木人桩的边门和打不正的角度; 如果对方比较弱, 就进入中门; 如果对方比较强, 就进入边门.

Think five petals of the plum flower:
- Mind keeps thinking
- Eyes keep observing
- Hands keep searching and seizing
- Body remains animated
- Feet keep evading

梅花的五个花瓣:
- 心神继续思考.
- 眼睛继续观察.
- 手继续找和抓.
- 身依然动画.
- 脚保持逃避.

Be opportunistic and unpredictable remembering the six harmonies of external and internal work:
- Six Externals: Fists, eyes, arms, steps, body, strength.
- Six Internals: Skill, tactics, boldness, swiftness, fierceness,

practical.

别失机会和变幻莫测. 记住六合内和外功:

- 　　　六个外功: 拳头，眼睛，手臂，马步，身体，力量。
- 　　　六个内功: 技术，战术，气魄，迅捷，凶猛，实用。

One should not forget and should endeavor to train the 18 Points of Internal Work in each technique when playing the dummy skills. Without having ingrained the principles, correct body posture, and fundamental hand skills, dummy work will not be useful or fruitful. If you know the Southern Mantis principles and fundamentals then any apparatus will become your dummy. Read my book "Eighteen Buddha Hands."

你不应该忘记，应该努力训练木人桩时，训练每一个手法的18点内功. 如果没有采用原理，正确的身体姿势，和基本手法，训练木人桩是不会有成果. 如果您知道南螳螂原理和基本原理则，任何培训设备将成为你的木人桩. 读我的书"十八佛手"。

Understand and master each movement before moving to the next one.

理解和熟练每一个动作才去下一个

Keep in mind that Southern Mantis uses three bridges which you may train on the wooden man. First bridge strengthens the limbs and matches strength by using the superior crushing bridge with slight angles and deflections. Second bridge is not designed to strengthen the limbs but to train you to gain from one superior position to another by taking up the most suitable position through footwork and using second hand to borrow force. Third bridge requires light body skill, agility, and footwork to simply not be where the opponent is striking - he always finds an empty target - you are no longer where he thought to strike when he arrives.

请记住，南螳螂使用三桥与你可以训练在木人桩. 第一桥加强四肢和用力对力破碎力的小角度和偏转. 第二桥训练你加强你的位置以步法和用第二段螳螂手来借力. 第三桥需要轻功，灵活和步法来偏转对方的攻击. 对方总是打空虚.

In qigong one refines the audible breath to inaudible. In Southern Mantis the four word secret of float, sink, swallow and spit is first visibly large and small, short and tall, before refined into one economy of motion that does not need exaggeration. Do what only is necessary. In playing the wooden man dummy the trainee who makes the noisiest movements while executing the dummy skills does not make the best use of it.

在气功，你提炼呼吸变无声。在南螳螂, 浮, 沉, 吞, 吐, 开始时动作很大和夸张. 慢慢提炼变成动作经济，没有夸张动作. 只做必要的动作。在训炼木人桩，谁炼最大声没有经济动作.

Use the shoulder, hip, and knee moving in unison to deliver whole body power at once. Shake up the wooden man, your opponent, with whole body power. Hand and foot together arrive intently on the target at once with whole body power.

用肩，髋，和膝一次提供全身力量。用全身力量打木人桩或对方. 用全身力量, 手和脚一起到达目标.

After you have by rote the wooden dummy routine, then train it is a shadowboxing routine, without the aid.

你学习木人桩套路之后，然后训练那个套路在空中，别用木人桩.

METHODS OF DUMMY TRAINING
木人桩训练方法

Three Methods:
• Train on the dummy to develop the basic skills, proper form, use of footwork, eye hand coordination, etc.
• Practice the applications with a live partner in order to learn rooting, feeling hand, and target practice.
• Practice the dummy set beating the air as a form, shadowboxing, solo training.

三种方法:
•   训练木人桩于熟练基本功，正确套路，步法, 眼手协调等等。
•   跟真人练习用途，以学习生根，摸手和目标练习.
•   练习木人桩套路在空中，练习手法在空中, 单人训练.

This is broken down into three categories:
• Hard (Crushing) Bridge- Blatant Attacks
• Soft (Borrowing Force) Bridge - confrontation and counter attacks
• Evasive (Neutralizing) Bridge and maneuvers

这个可以分为三类:
•   硬桥（破碎） - 明显的攻击
•   软桥（借力） - 对抗与反击
• 逃避（抵消） - 移动

DUMMY BENEFIT
木人桩的好处

Techniques that are considered dangerous, even lethal, can be practiced without the fear of maiming your partner. You may train as if facing a "real" opponent.
手法认为是危险的，甚至致命的，可以安全在木人桩练不怕打伤人.
你可以训练像"真正"面对对方.

DUMMY TRAINING GOAL
木人桩的训练目标

Use the dummy, in absence of a real person, to refine the horse, posture and fundamental skills which you can then use when you have a live partner. This kind of dummy work will help you to move from the conscious to the instinctive level of training. Read the "Eighteen Buddha Hands" book to understand intuitive training.

没有真人训练，可以用木人桩来提炼马步，姿势和基本功. 然后你就可以使用当你有真人训练. 这种木人桩训练可以帮助你从意识转移到直觉的反应. 读"十八佛手"来了解训练直觉的反应.

PREREQUISITES

Before reading this book you should at least have studied:

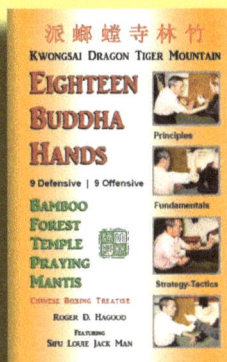

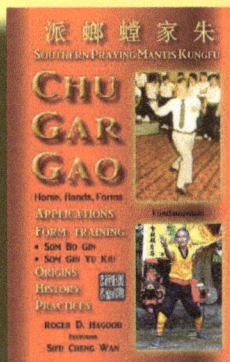

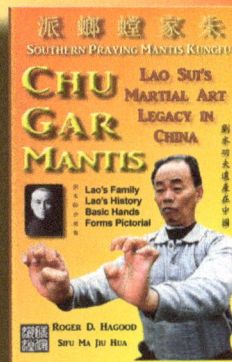

Amazon, Barnes and Noble, Books-A-Million

槍历史 ABOUT POLE TECHNIQUES

I don't emphasize classical weapons in my teaching, rather we focus on becoming skillful at the boxing basics. The saying is, "if the hand is skillful, anything one picks up becomes a weapon".

Whether you call them cudgels, staffs, or poles, sticks are more of a traditional relic than a practical weapon of defense, in our urban societies. They are less lethal than knives or guns but still can cause deadly blunt trauma, broken bones, and serious bruising.

Sticks (gun) yet have a prominent role in a traditional Chinese martial arts school. Usually the first and foremost weapon taught in any traditional martial arts school, the staff is known as "king or father" of the four major weapons, along with the qiang (spear), dao (broadsword), and the jian (sword).

One might say the reason why this weapon precedes others is because its techniques create a foundation for training all other weapons.

Five blocking techniques are:
- circular block
- leg block
- vertical block
- outside block
- horizontal block

Seven striking techniques are:
- the downward strike
- straight thrust
- uppercut
- figure eight striking
- overhead clouding
- diagonal strike
- the horizontal strike

Benefits of Staff Play
- Increased Power / Strength
- Extension of Power Reaching to Fingertips
- Extended Distance / Range in Attack - Defense

Benefits of Two Person Staff Play:
- Body control and coordination in Attack and Defense
- Timing (more important than speed)
- Accuracy in Vital Point Attack and Defense

Generally, a staff should be equal to one's own height, but short sticks to eyebrow height and long poles up to four meters are not uncommon. Both wood and metal sticks may be employed and are found in many variations such as swinging sectioned staffs, club heads, and iron toothed heads.

陈建明师傅

YELLOW OX POLE

Many pole forms, single and two man, exist. Some routines are short with as few as a dozen movements and some are as long as 108. The Hakka Mantis form shown herein is only some 17 movements.

The correct name of this form when translated is more like, Yellow Ox Entering Battle. I will refer to it as simply, Yellow Ox Pole.

Single and Double tip play is employed. The striking tip of the staff is called the "pole head" in Chinese. Hakka Pole is usually single end play and this Yellow Ox Pole form herein, is single end play.

Besides the blocking and striking attributes listed above, the Hakka pole is usually concerned with striking below the waist and especially the toes. One can see "chicken pecking rice" in the succession of ground strikes chasing and striking the opponent's feet.

Lam Sang's first and second generation Kwongsai Mantis disciples in the 1950s-60s, USA, played both single end pole and double end.

I only offer this glimpse of the simple but rare, Chu Mantis Yellow Ox Pole form for your perusal. It's a pictorial, not instructional. Perhaps, I'll try to release further details and instruction on a DVD, in the future.

Opening Posture 1

YELLOW OX POLE

Five blocking techniques are:

- circular block
- leg block
- vertical block
- outside block
- horizontal block

Seven striking techniques are:

- the downward strike
- straight thrust
- uppercut
- figure eight striking
- overhead clouding
- diagonal strike
- the horizontal strike

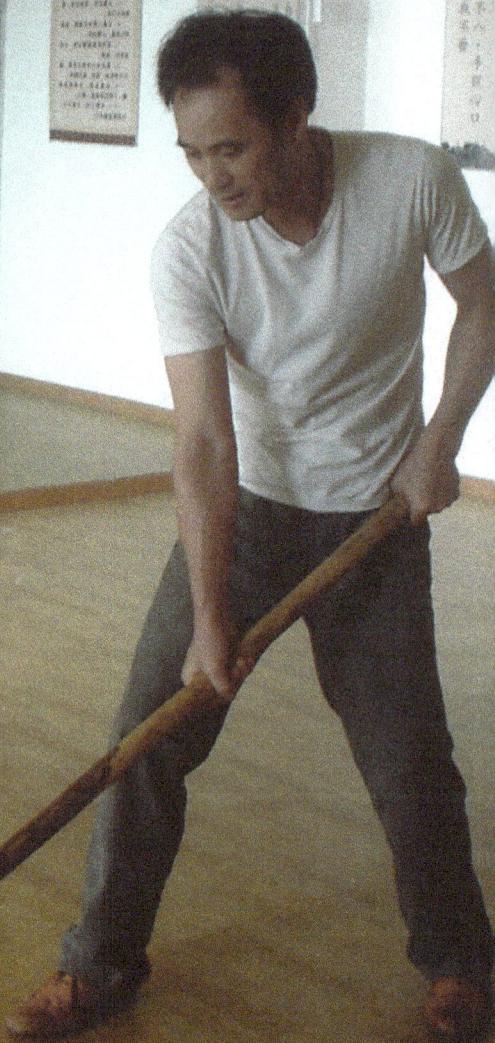

2

Online Video: www.southmantis.com

陈建明師傅

YELLOW OX POLE

Five blocking techniques are:
- circular block
- leg block
- vertical block
- outside block
- horizontal block

Seven striking techniques are:
- the downward strike
- straight thrust
- uppercut
- figure eight striking
- overhead clouding
- diagonal strike
- the horizontal strike

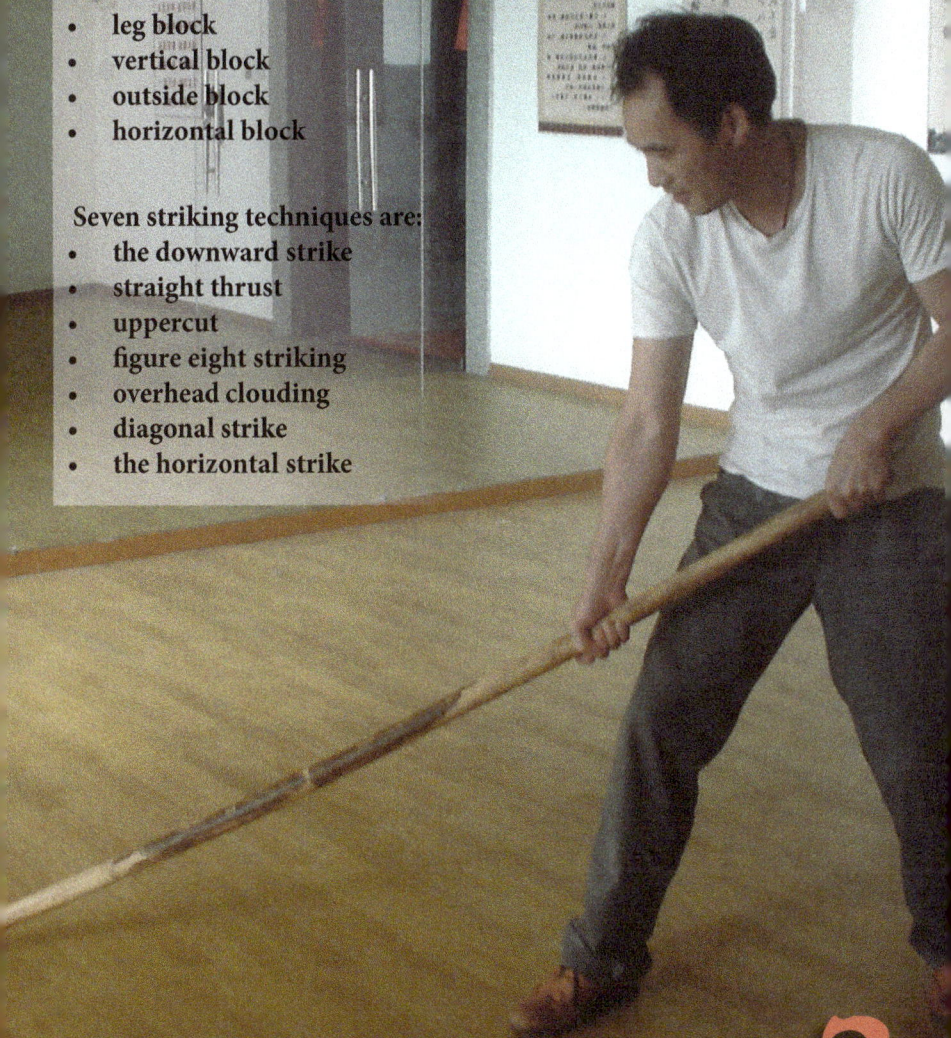

3

YELLOW OX POLE

Five blocking techniques are:

- circular block
- leg block
- vertical block
- outside block
- horizontal block

Seven striking techniques are:

- the downward strike
- straight thrust
- uppercut
- figure eight striking
- overhead clouding
- diagonal strike
- the horizontal strike

4

Online Video: www.southmantis.com

陈建明师傅

YELLOW OX POLE

Five blocking techniques are:

- circular block
- leg block
- vertical block
- outside block
- horizontal block

Seven striking techniques are:

- the downward strike
- straight thrust
- uppercut
- figure eight striking
- overhead clouding
- diagonal strike
- the horizontal strike

5

Online Video: www.southmantis.com

YELLOW OX POLE

Five blocking techniques are:
- circular block
- leg block
- vertical block
- outside block
- horizontal block

Seven striking techniques are:
- the downward strike
- straight thrust
- uppercut
- figure eight striking
- overhead clouding
- diagonal strike
- the horizontal strike

6

YELLOW OX POLE

Five blocking techniques are:

- circular block
- leg block
- vertical block
- outside block
- horizontal block

Seven striking techniques are:

- the downward strike
- straight thrust
- uppercut
- figure eight striking
- overhead clouding
- diagonal strike
- the horizontal strike

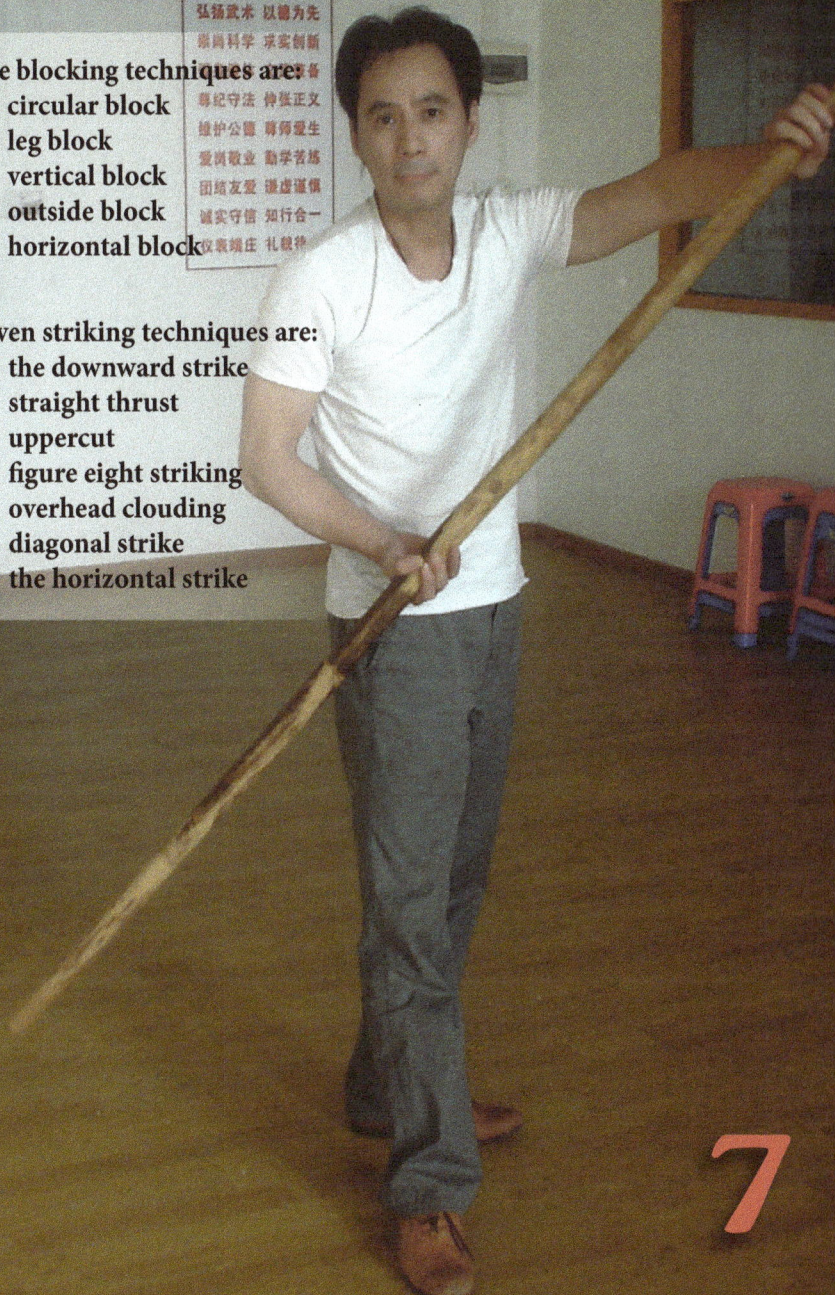

7

Online Video: www.southmantis.com

YELLOW OX POLE

Five blocking techniques are:

- circular block
- leg block
- vertical block
- outside block
- horizontal block

Seven striking techniques are:

- the downward strike
- straight thrust
- uppercut
- figure eight striking
- overhead clouding
- diagonal strike
- the horizontal strike

8

YELLOW OX POLE

陈建明師傅

Five blocking techniques are:
* circular block
* leg block
* vertical block
* outside block
* horizontal block

Seven striking techniques are:
* the downward strike
* straight thrust
* uppercut
* figure eight striking
* overhead clouding
* diagonal strike
* the horizontal strike

9

Online Video: www.southmantis.com

YELLOW OX POLE

Five blocking techniques are:

- circular block
- leg block
- vertical block
- outside block
- horizontal block

Seven striking techniques are:

- the downward strike
- straight thrust
- uppercut
- figure eight striking
- overhead clouding
- diagonal strike
- the horizontal strike

10

Online Video: www.southmantis.com

陈建明师傅

YELLOW OX POLE

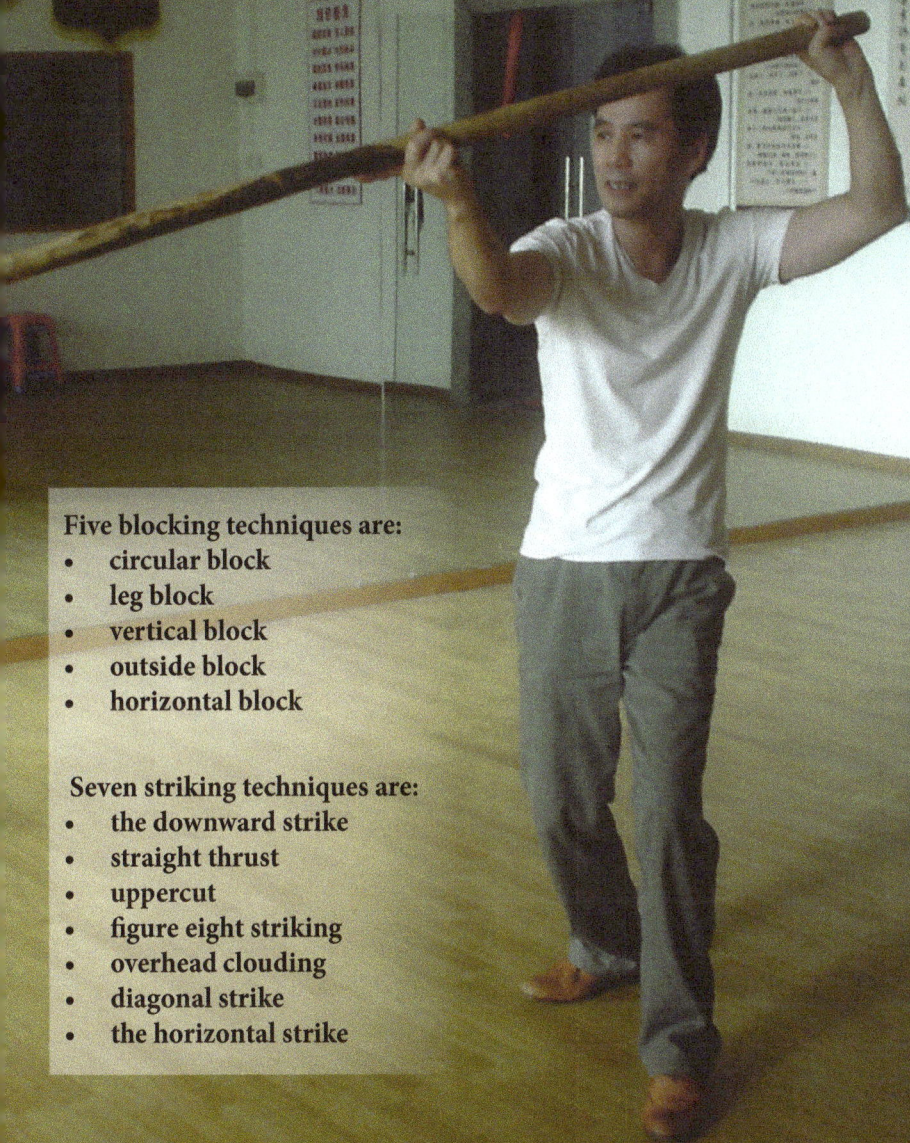

Five blocking techniques are:
- circular block
- leg block
- vertical block
- outside block
- horizontal block

Seven striking techniques are:
- the downward strike
- straight thrust
- uppercut
- figure eight striking
- overhead clouding
- diagonal strike
- the horizontal strike

11

Online Video: www.southmantis.com

YELLOW OX POLE

Five blocking techniques are:
- circular block
- leg block
- vertical block
- outside block
- horizontal block

Seven striking techniques are:
- the downward strike
- straight thrust
- uppercut
- figure eight striking
- overhead clouding
- diagonal strike
- the horizontal strike

12

Online Video: www.southmantis.com

陈建明師傅

YELLOW OX POLE

Five blocking techniques are:
- circular block
- leg block
- vertical block
- outside block
- horizontal block

Seven striking techniques are:
- the downward strike
- straight thrust
- uppercut
- figure eight striking
- overhead clouding
- diagonal strike
- the horizontal strike

13

Online Video: www.southmantis.com

YELLOW OX POLE

Five blocking techniques are:
- circular block
- leg block
- vertical block
- outside block
- horizontal block

Seven striking techniques are:
- the downward strike
- straight thrust
- uppercut
- figure eight striking
- overhead clouding
- diagonal strike
- the horizontal strike

14

Online Video: www.southmantis.com

陈建明師傅

YELLOW OX POLE

Five blocking techniques are:
- circular block
- leg block
- vertical block
- outside block
- horizontal block

Seven striking techniques are:
- the downward strike
- straight thrust
- uppercut
- figure eight striking
- overhead clouding
- diagonal strike
- the horizontal strike

15

Online Video: www.southmantis.com

YELLOW OX POLE

Five blocking techniques are:
- circular block
- leg block
- vertical block
- outside block
- horizontal block

Seven striking techniques are:
- the downward strike
- straight thrust
- uppercut
- figure eight striking
- overhead clouding
- diagonal strike
- the horizontal strike

16

陈建明师傅

YELLOW OX POLE

Five blocking techniques are:
- circular block
- leg block
- vertical block
- outside block
- horizontal block

Seven striking techniques are:
- the downward strike
- straight thrust
- uppercut
- figure eight striking
- overhead clouding
- diagonal strike
- the horizontal strike

17

Online Video: www.southmantis.com

YELLOW OX POLE

1

Prepare
Application

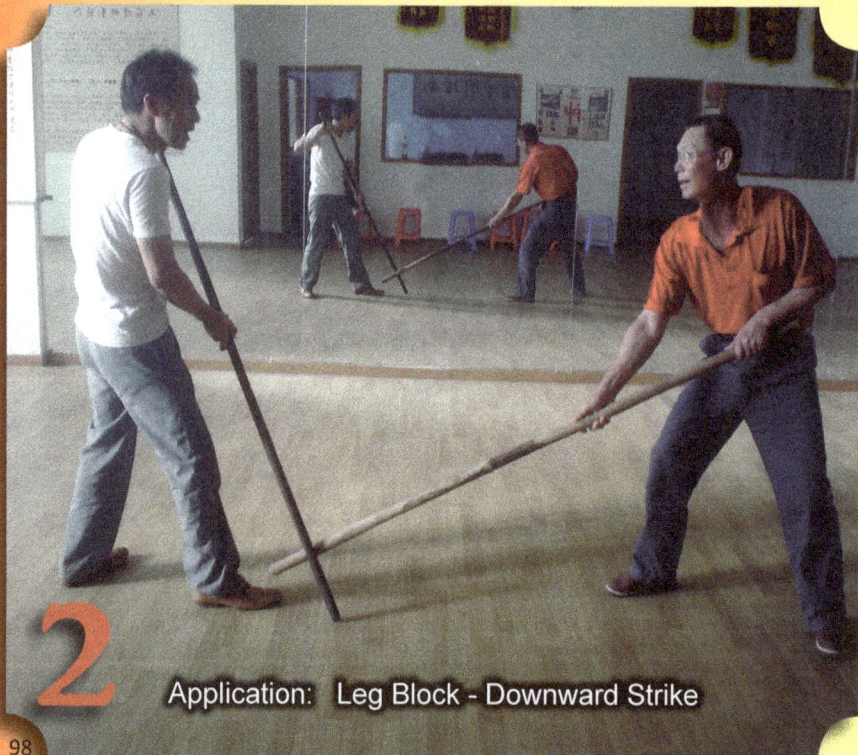

2

Application:　Leg Block - Downward Strike

YELLOW OX POLE

谢添胜师傅

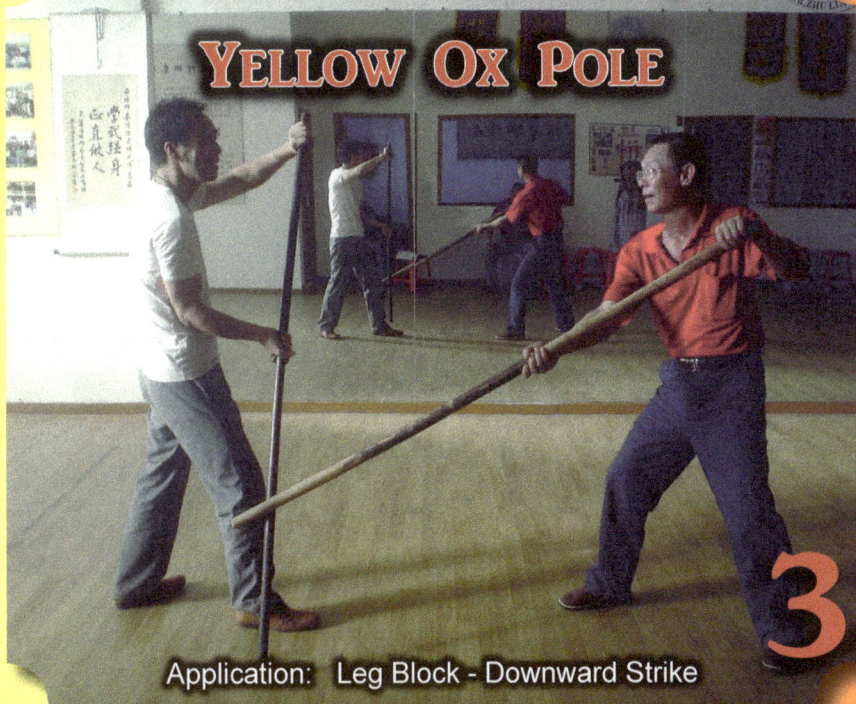

3

Application: Leg Block - Downward Strike

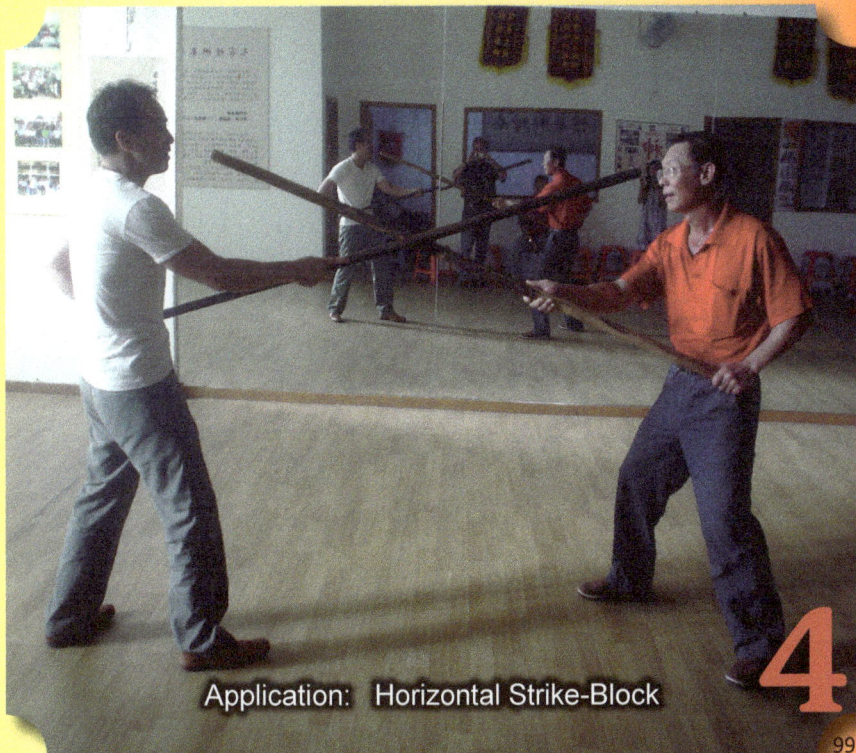

4

Application: Horizontal Strike-Block

YELLOW OX POLE

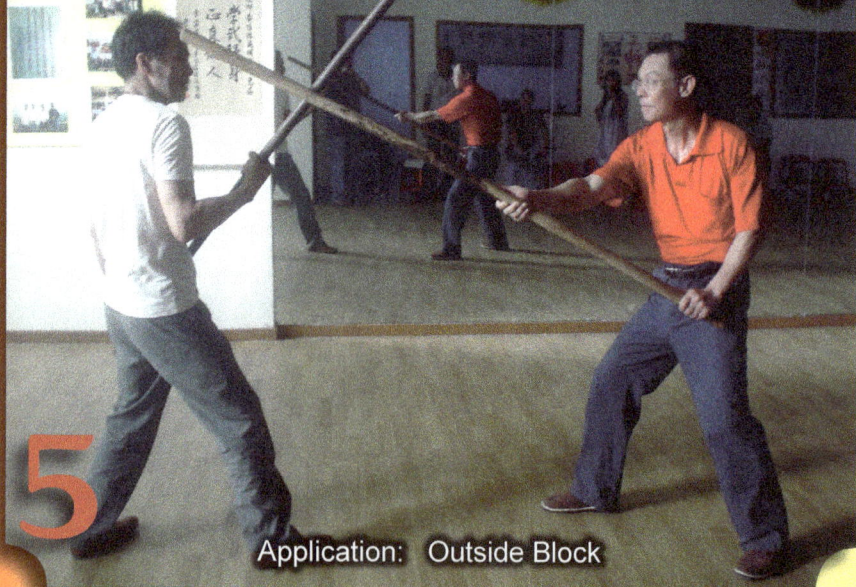

5

Application: Outside Block

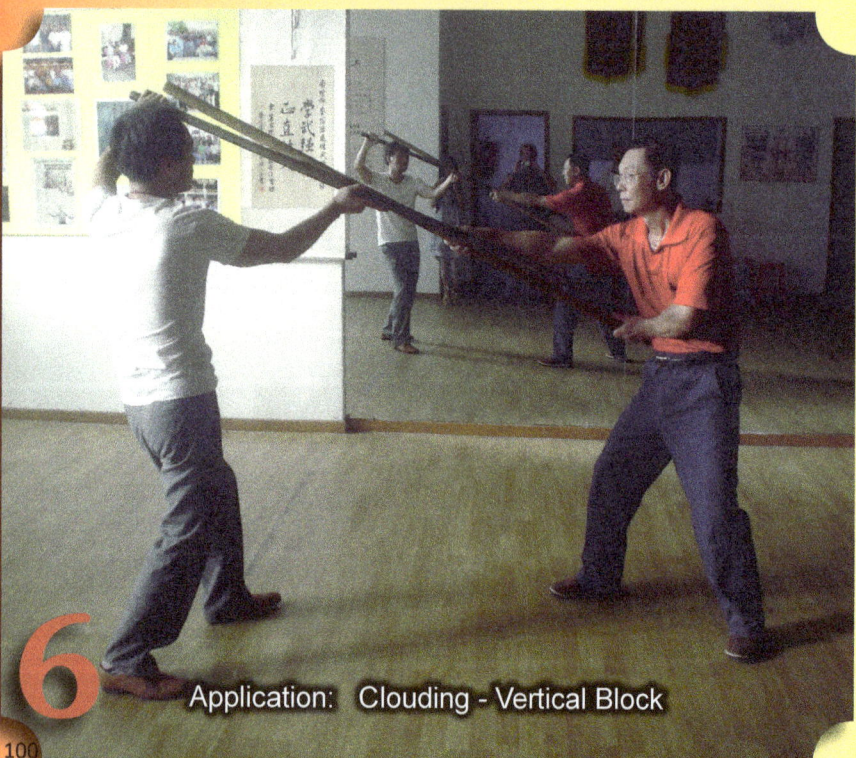

6

Application: Clouding - Vertical Block

謝添勝師傅

YELLOW OX POLE

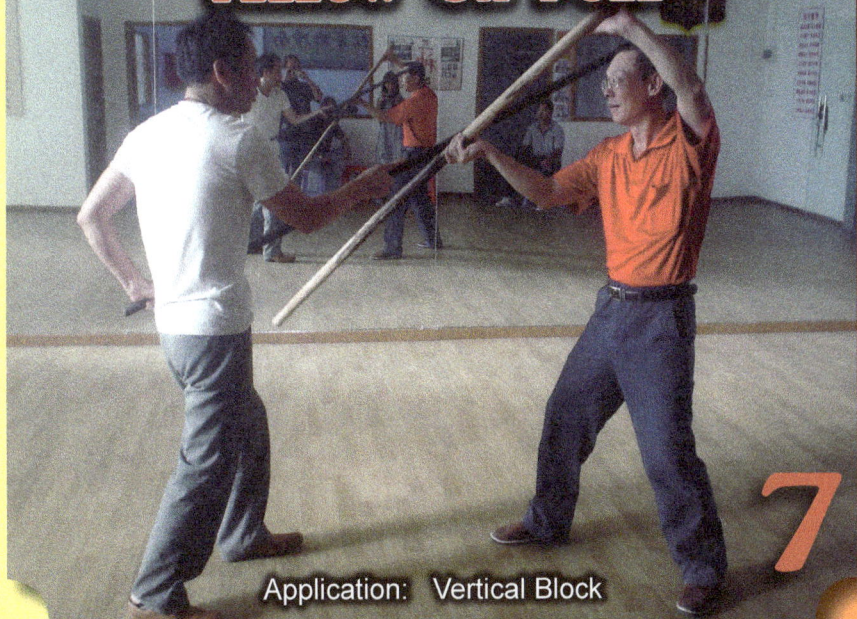

7

Application: Vertical Block

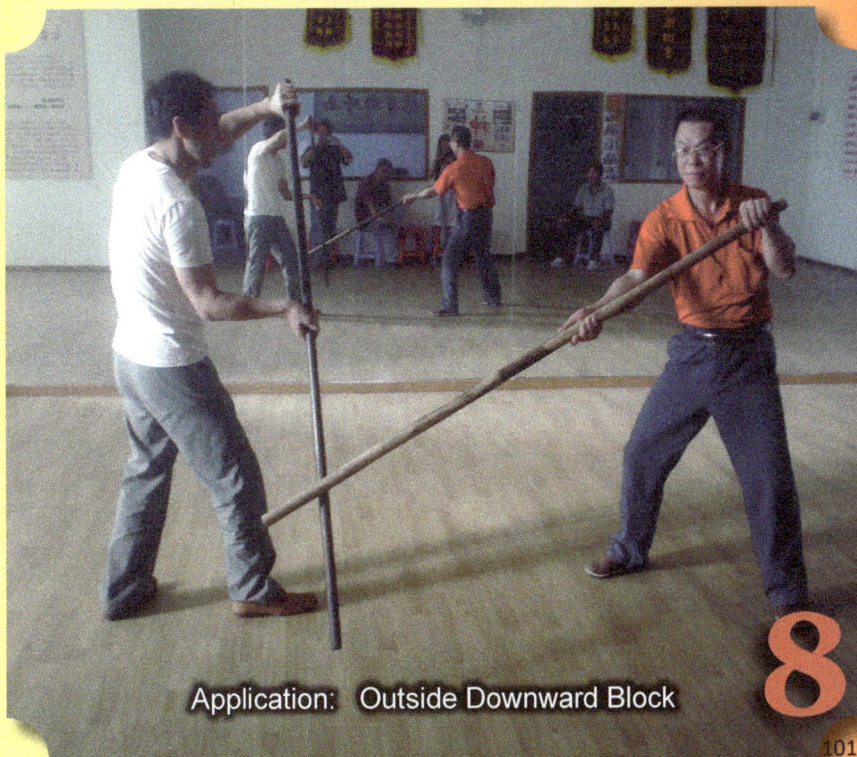

8

Application: Outside Downward Block

YELLOW OX POLE

9

Application: Thrust - Vertical Block

10

Application: Clouding

谢添胜师傅

YELLOW OX POLE

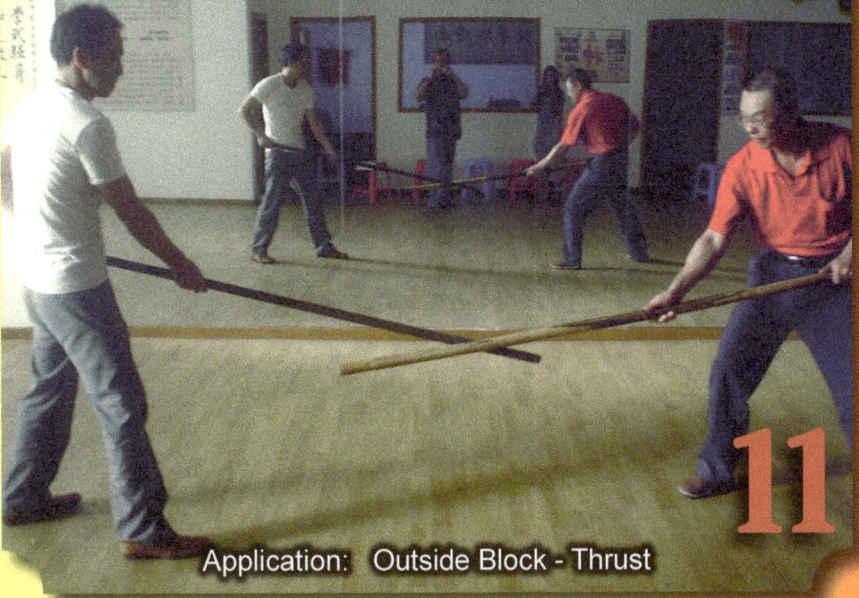

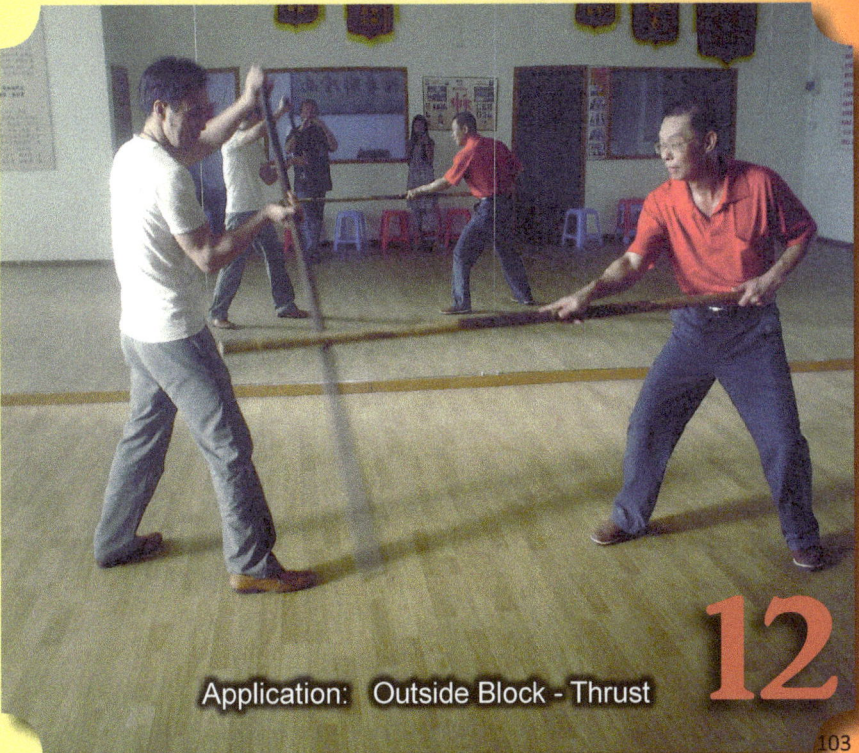

11

Application: Outside Block - Thrust

12

Application: Outside Block - Thrust

About Dui Jong Paired Training

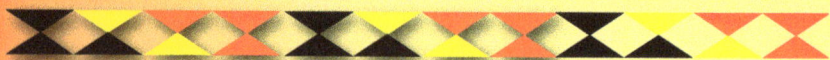

Dui Jong has become a catch-phrase for any kind of paired training, two person training. Commonly, in Hakka Mantis we say "two man" training or forms. Of course, it isn't proper English. "Two Man" is common and more of a direct English-Chinese translation. Like the Hakka Mantis saying, "One must Cheat the other's power". Cheating is not an exact translation but we could hear the elders using "Chinglish" to say "cheat" his power.

DUI JONG PAIRED TRAINING

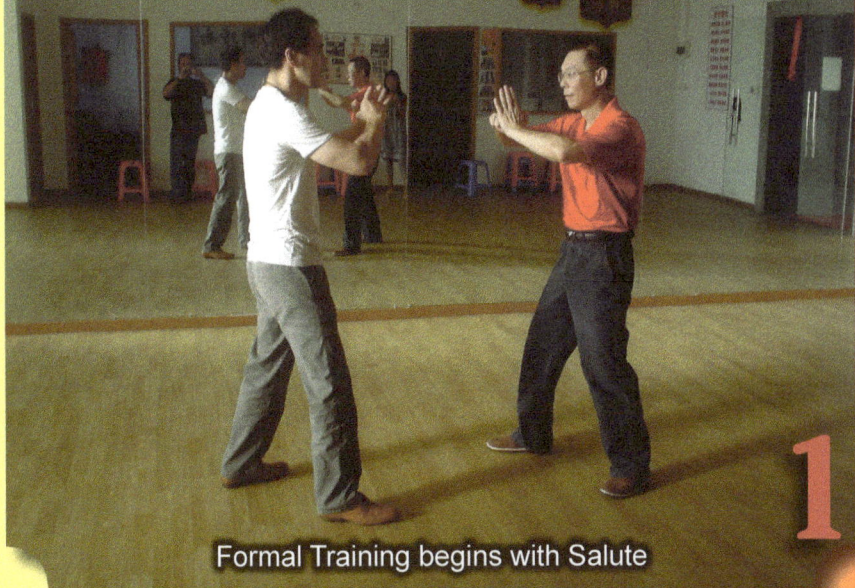

Formal Training begins with Salute

1

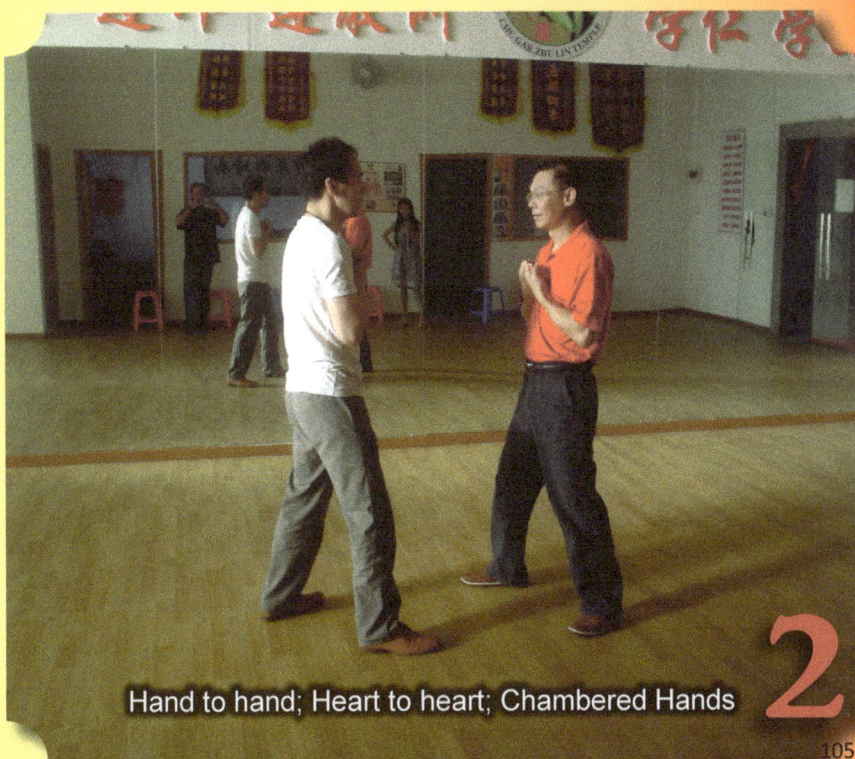

Hand to hand; Heart to heart; Chambered Hands

2

105

DUI JONG PAIRED TRAINING

陈建明師傅

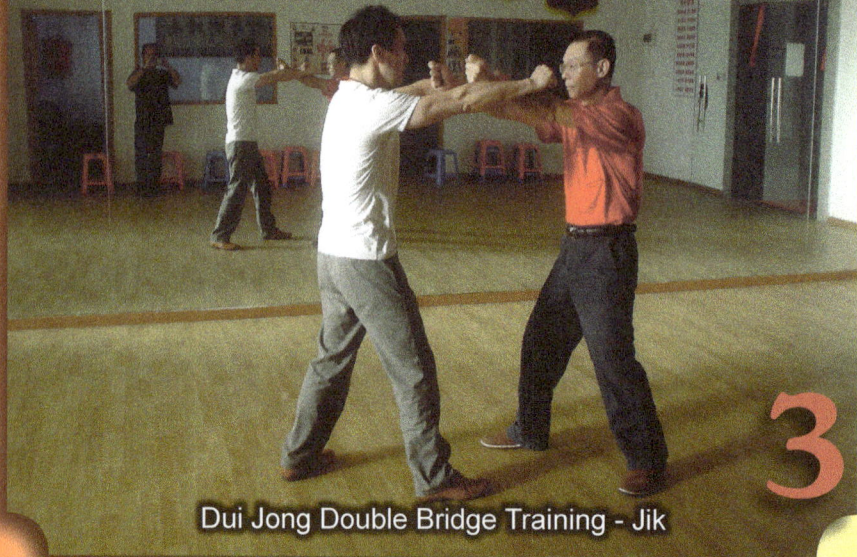

3

Dui Jong Double Bridge Training - Jik

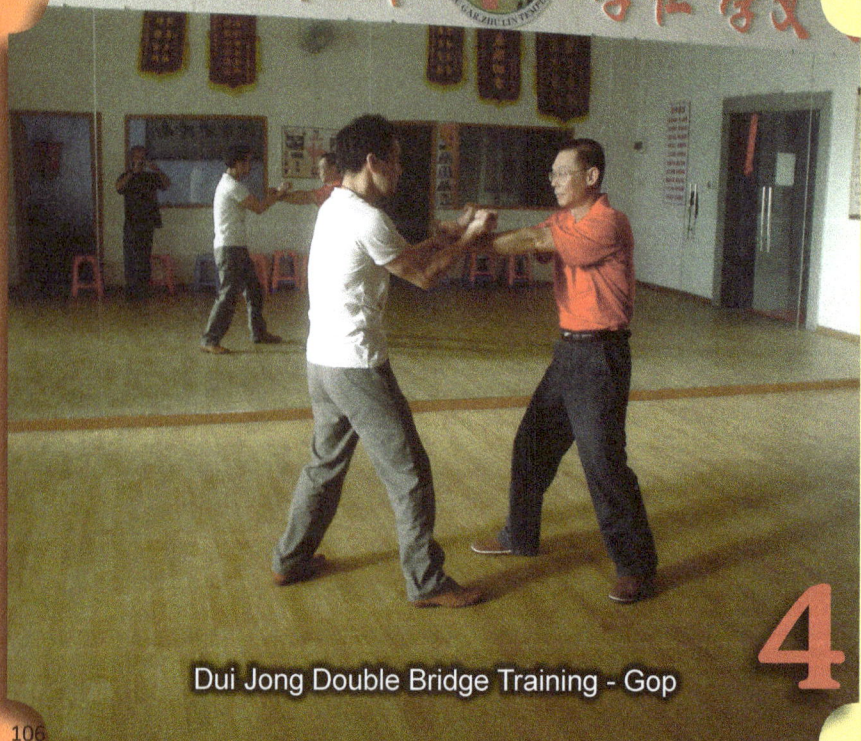

4

Dui Jong Double Bridge Training - Gop

106

DUI JONG PAIRED TRAINING

谢添胜師傅

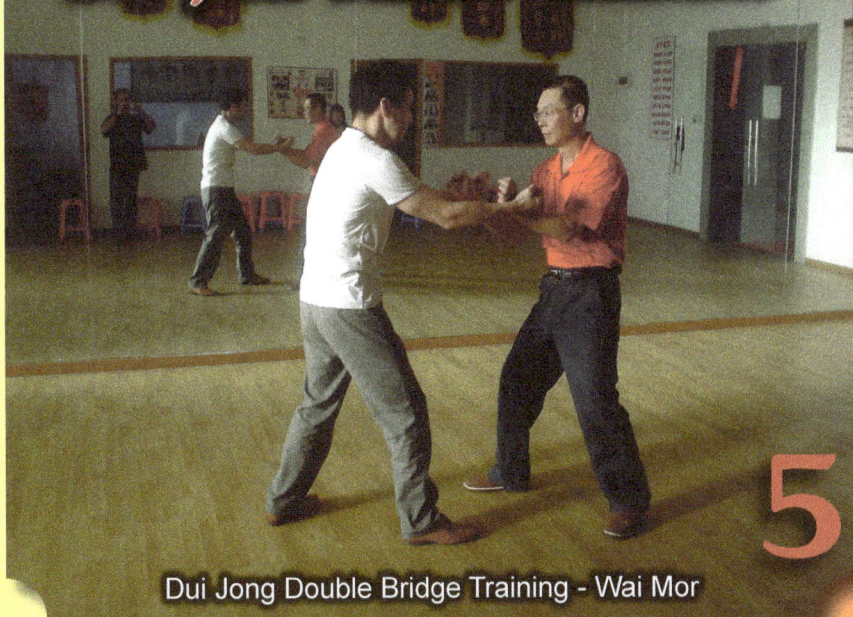

5

Dui Jong Double Bridge Training - Wai Mor

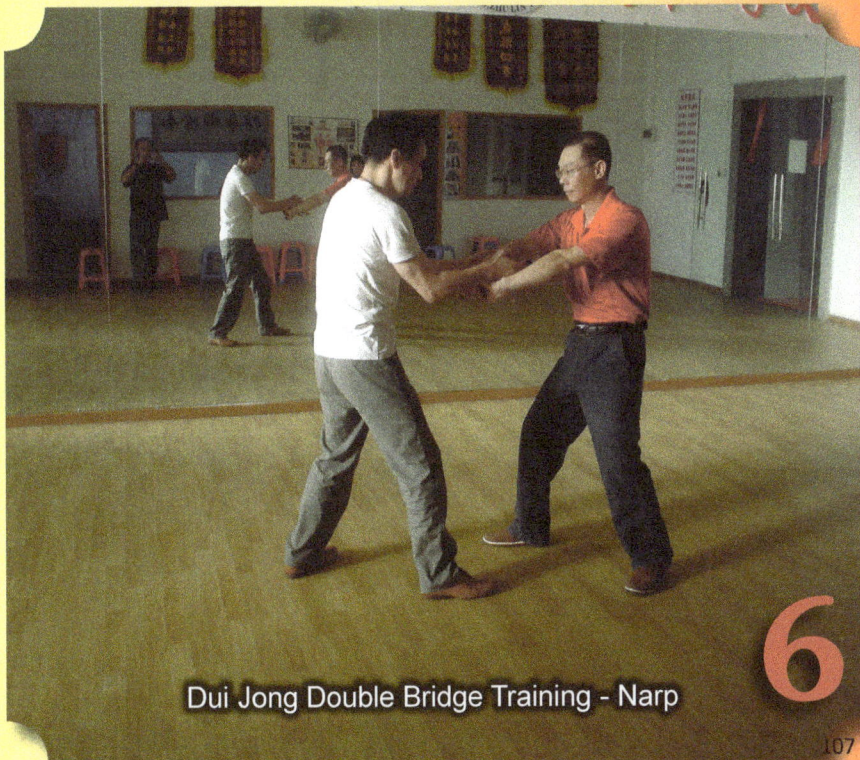

6

Dui Jong Double Bridge Training - Narp

107

DUI JONG PAIRED TRAINING

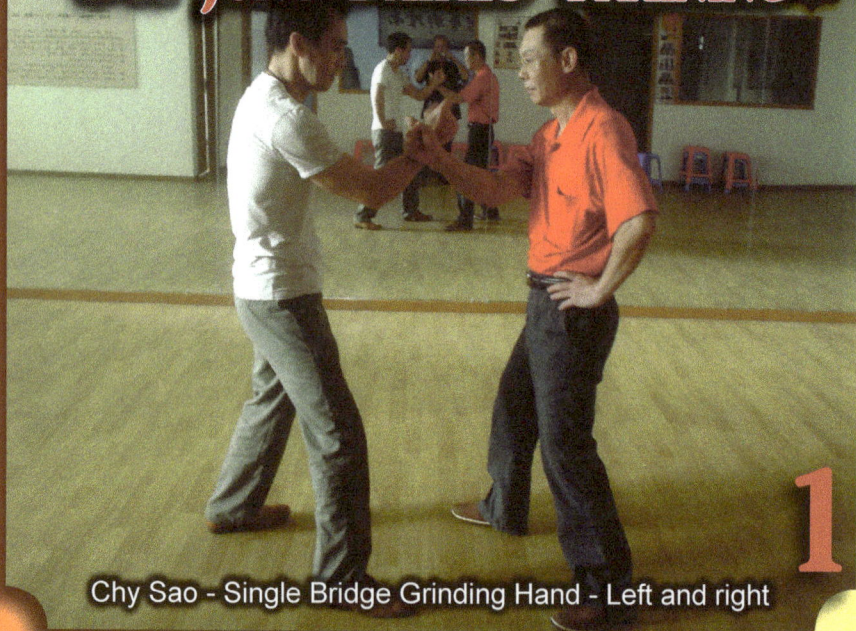

Chy Sao - Single Bridge Grinding Hand - Left and right

1

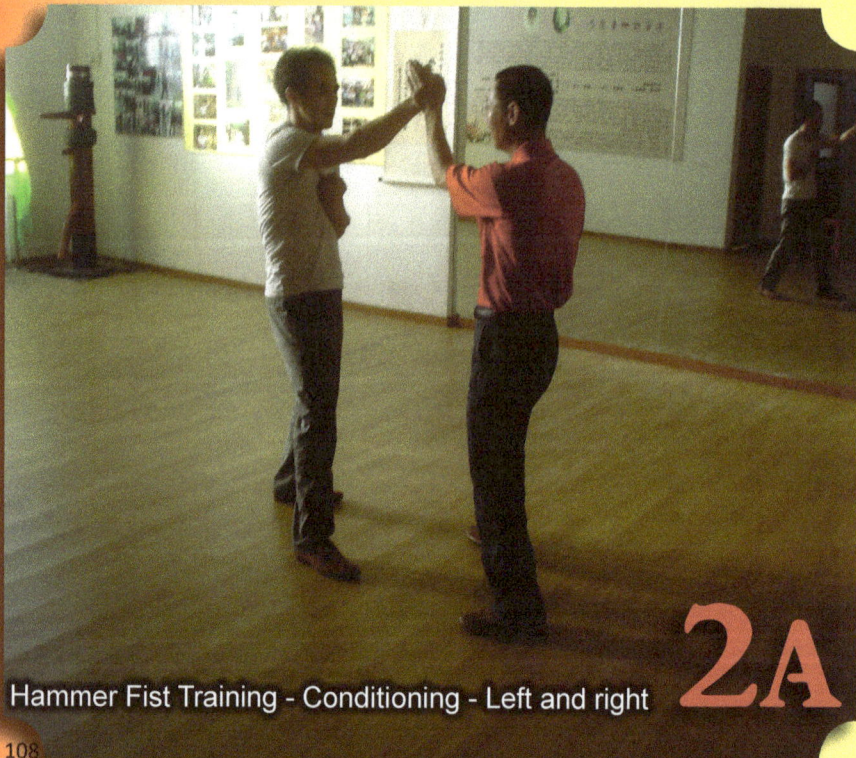

Hammer Fist Training - Conditioning - Left and right

2A

DUI JONG PAIRED TRAINING

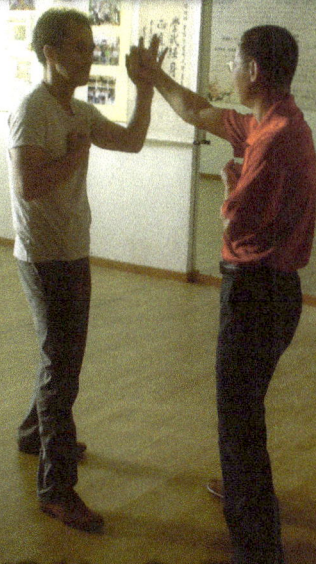

2B

Hammer Fist Training - Conditioning - Both Players

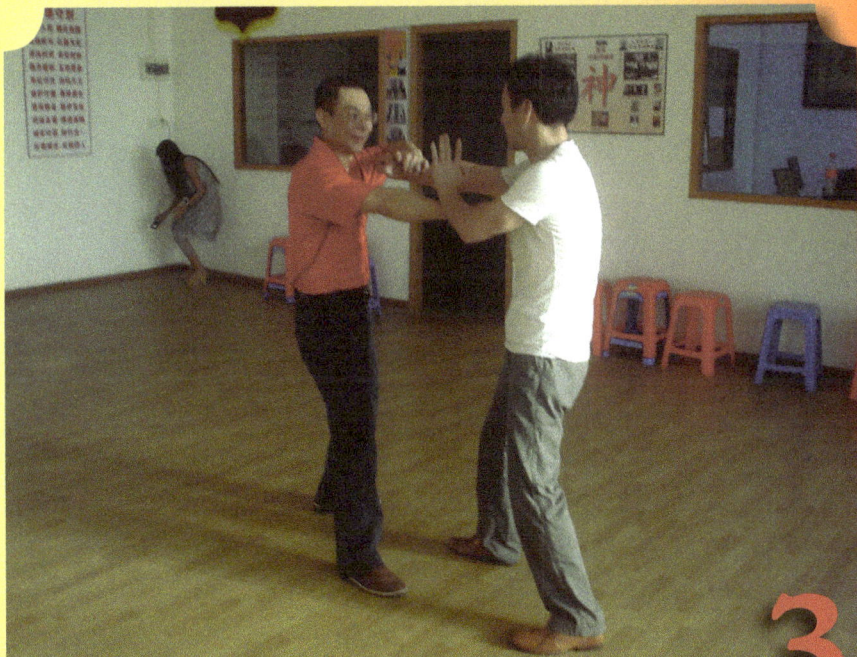

3

Man Dang Sao Dui Jong - Left and right; both players

Recap

On this book cover, we see the Yang Clan first generation Chu Gar, from Wong Fook Go and perhaps Lao Sui.

In 2013, the Yang Clan performed the Unicorn celebrations, in which I cooperated with Chen Jianming to open the first public school of Chu Gar, in Lao Sui's hometown. Chen Sifu is a descendent of Lao's second generation teaching.

Following the narrative of the Huizhou School opening, which included Li Tinloi and his followers of Yip Sui's "Chow Gar", I have introduced briefly the use of wooden man or wooden dummy and its limited role in training.

Futher, Chen Jianming Sifu, of the Huizhou clan, has recounted the 17 or so steps of the Yellow Ox Pole form. It is a single end Hakka Pole technique. Xie Tiansheng Sifu has participated in the applications of this pole form.

Moreover, Chen and Xie Sifus have demonstrated the four basic two man methods of Chu Gar, or Dui Jongs. Generally speaking, all the Chu Gar clans have these basic methods. The order shown is not the order usually trained. The methods in order may be:
1) Chy Sao - Single Bridge grinding hand or arms
2) Dui Jong - Double Bridge Training
3) Man Dang Sao Dui Jong - A peculiar simultaneous defense-offense; only found in Lam Sang's USA Kwongsai Mantis, not China Kwongsai Mantis; Sometimes the ending of Chu Gar single man forms, especially in Yip Sui's "Chow Gar"
4) Gow Choy Hammer Fist - Two man palm and fist conditioning

Read on now and join the Yang Clan of Chu Gar Mantis who descended from Yang Shou. Some say Yang Shou was a student of Wong Fook Go in Huiyang. We do know he was with Lao Sui in the 1920s / 30s in Hong Kong. Even some Kwongsai Mantis players have referred to Yang Shou as "Uncle".

Yang Style Chu Gar Mantis

History and Pictorial

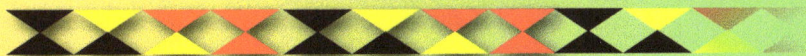

楊
式
朱
家

楊式朱家

Yang Style Chu Gar History & Pictorial

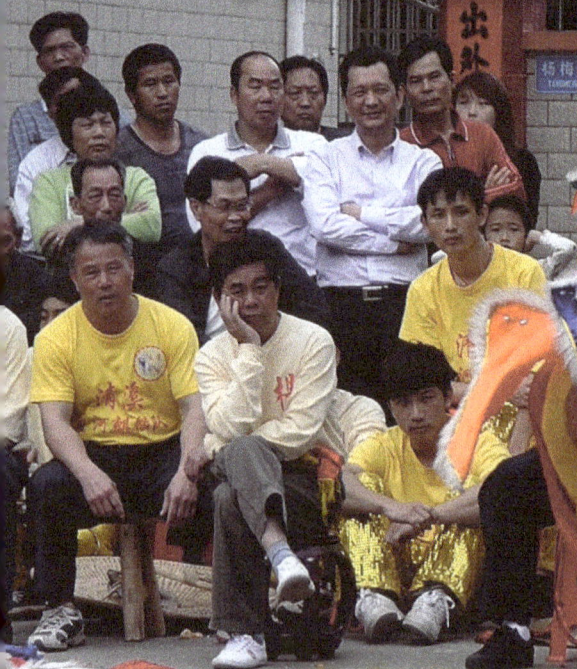

廣東省東莞市

Dongguan, Guangdong
Lao Sui's Kungfu Legacy in China

劉水功夫遺產在中國

112

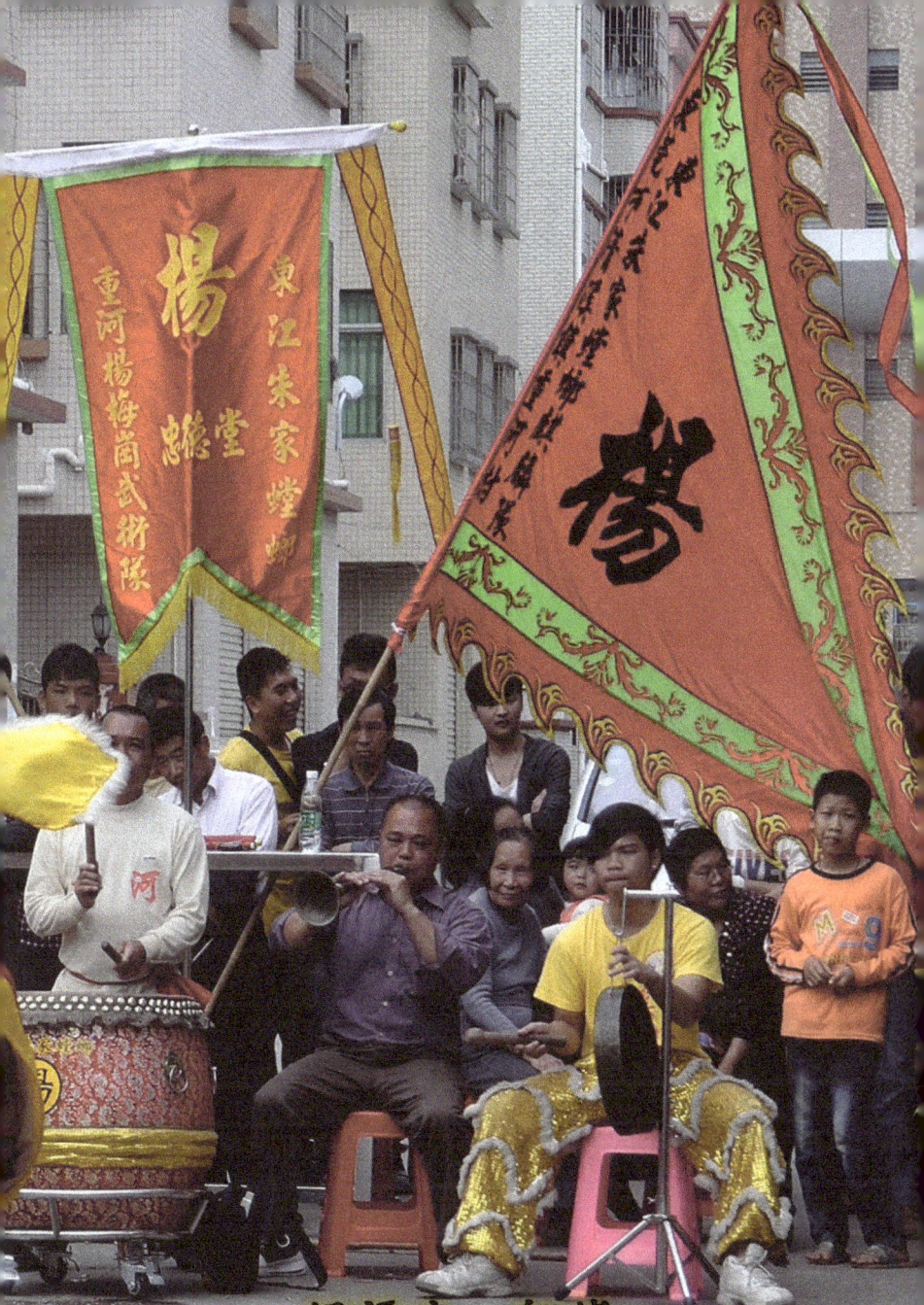

楊譚鹿　師傅

SIGONG YANG TANG LU

SIFU YANG WEI

楊維　師傅

清溪杨梅岗村

Qingxi Town
Yang Mei Gang Village

Home of the late
Chu Gar
Master Yang Shou

This photo shows the Headquarters of the Yang Clan Chu Gar Mantis in Qingxi Town, Dongguan, China.

都有杨式朱家螳螂从杨秀传下来。杨秀是刘水的第一代第子在香港20世纪30年；杨秀是气势不凡和神密莫测的人物。我甚至听说过一些江西竹林寺螳螂叫他"伯伯"。甚至在他的家乡没有现存的照片的他，但众所周知，在 1940 年代以后，他回到清溪、东莞市、他的家乡去世。杨秀教过五个好的徒弟，包括黄莱。黄莱出生于 1912 年，享年 96 岁。在东莞市的清溪，从那天至今都有杨式朱家螳螂和客家麒麟文化都传自于黄莱之手。继续维护和促进杨式朱家螳螂和客家麒麟文化传输。杨式家族他们都是客家人。今天杨式的师公是杨谭鹿、杨维师傅，如上图所示。

杨维师傅接受他的第一个徒弟在 1981 年。开始的时候，他接受只有徒弟与他的氏族，杨，相同的姓氏，但后来决定接受所有人。

今天，他们的杨式朱家传输包括：马步、对钟、散手、三步剪、四门、六门、八门、棍、客家麒麟文化。事实上，2013年当我RDH，配合陈建明师傅在惠州，刘水家乡开第一个朱家螳螂武馆是杨维他们的麒麟团对陪我们一起庆祝活动。

我计划出版一本新书，详述这个宗族，在不久的将来。我将在即将到来的客家螳螂我比较分析包括杨氏族。有客家螳螂流派异同，当理解，提高能力，在拳击比赛中的。一点相似之处是乞丐手的姿势。

English translation on the following page

All the people above, of the Yang Clan Chu Gar Mantis, descend from Yang Shou, a first generation disciple of Lao Sui, in 1920s/30s Hong Kong. Yang Shou was a mysterious and powerful figure in Chu Gar and Hakka Mantis. I have even heard some in Kwongsai Mantis call him "uncle." There are no extant photos of him, even in his hometown, but, it is known he returned to Qingxi, Dongguan, China, his hometown, in the 1940s, and passed.

He, Yang Shou, taught five good students, including Wang Lai. Wang Lai was born in 1912 and died, at 96 years old.

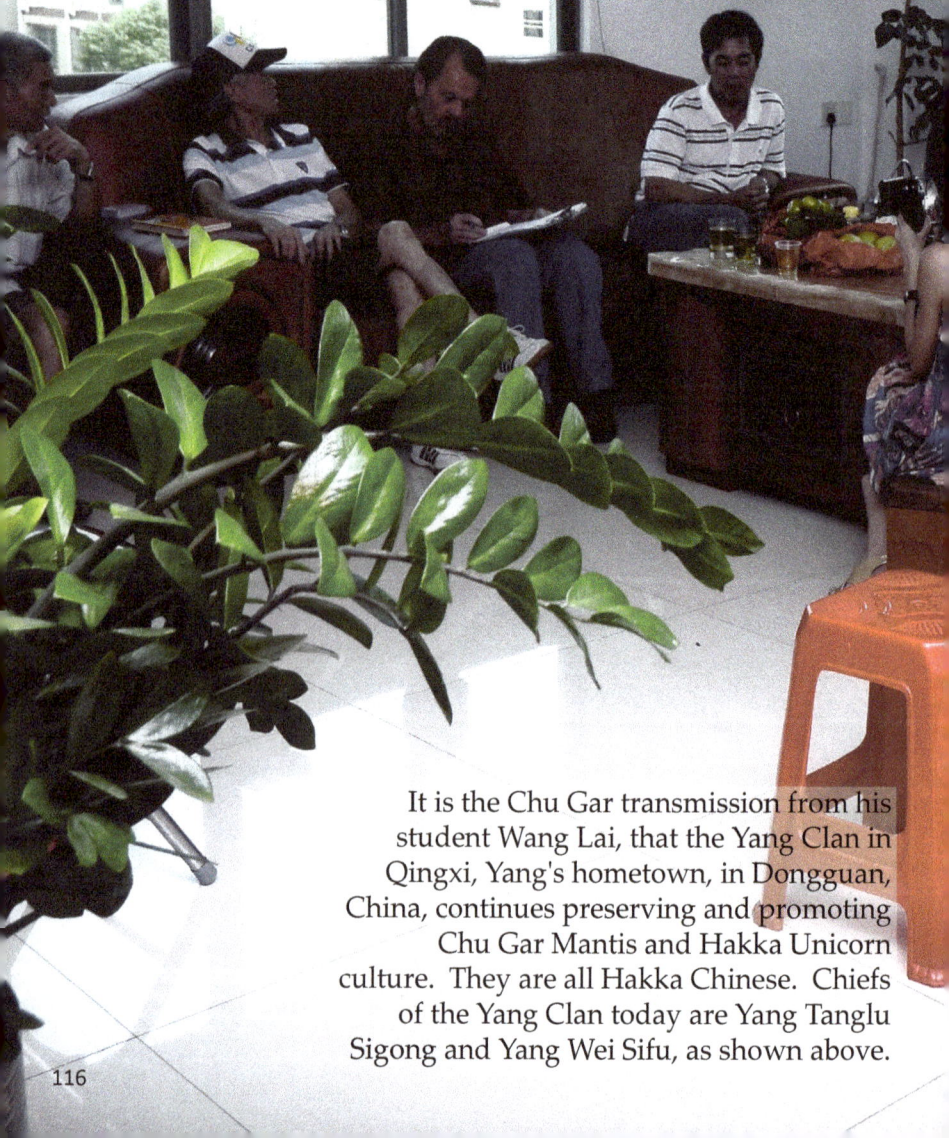

It is the Chu Gar transmission from his student Wang Lai, that the Yang Clan in Qingxi, Yang's hometown, in Dongguan, China, continues preserving and promoting Chu Gar Mantis and Hakka Unicorn culture. They are all Hakka Chinese. Chiefs of the Yang Clan today are Yang Tanglu Sigong and Yang Wei Sifu, as shown above.

Yang Wei Sifu accepted his first student, in 1981. In the beginning, he accepted only students with the same surname as his clan, Yang, but later decided to accept any and all.

Today, their Chu Gar transmission includes, horse, two man dui jong, san shou basics, forms Som Bo Gin, Four Gate, Six Gate, Eight Gate, Staff, and Hakka Unicorn culture. In fact, when I, RDH, cooperated with Chen Jianming Sifu last year to open the first public Chu Gar School, in Huizhou, Lao Sui's hometown, it was Yang Wei Sifu's clan who performed the Unicorn celebrations.

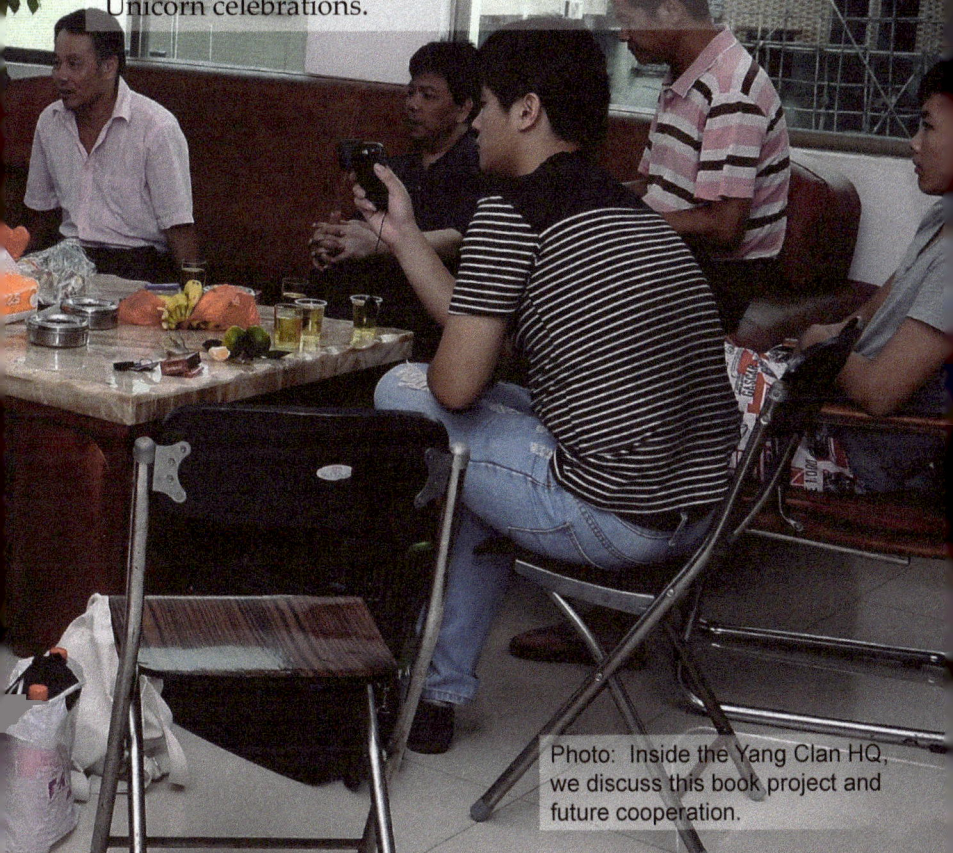

Photo: Inside the Yang Clan HQ, we discuss this book project and future cooperation.

I plan to release a book detailing this clan, in the near future. And I will be including the Yang Clan in my comparative analysis of Hakka Mantis upcoming. There are similarities and differences in the various Hakka Mantis Schools that when understood, increase one's ability in boxing. One similarity to all is the "Hat Yi Sao" Beggars Hand posture.

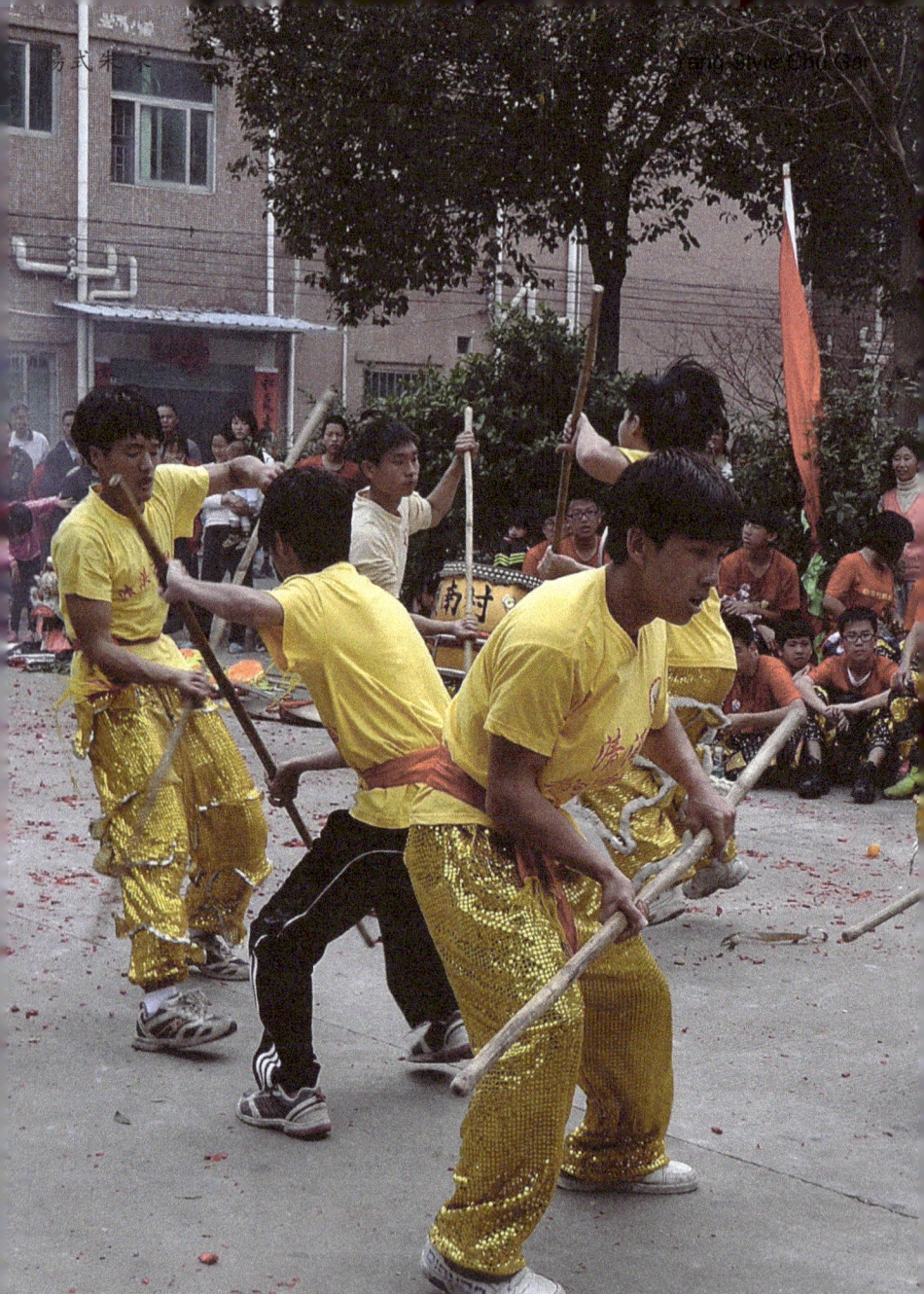

A traditional Chinese Kungfu expo, of the Hakka people, usually begins with a Unicorn dancing several skits and is followed by the youth of the group showing shadowboxing and paired demonstrations of empty hand and weapons sets. Afterwards, all esteemed guests of the event are invited to demonstrate their boxing, before the adult members of the host clan show their hand youngest to oldest, with the final performance always being the host Sifu.

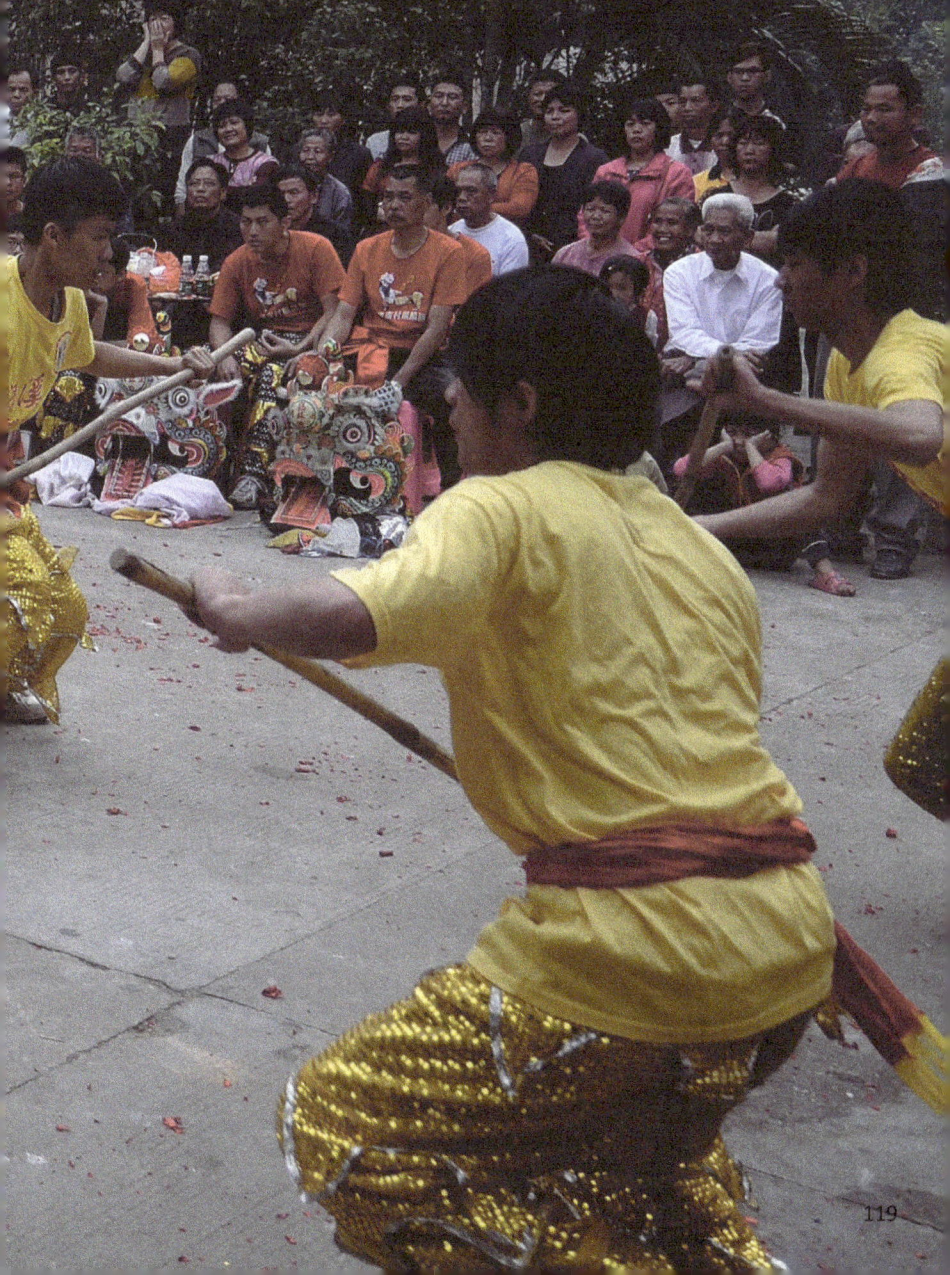

YANG STYLE CHU GAR YOUTH BOXERS & UNICORN TROUPE

YANG CLAN
CHU GAR

楊式朱家

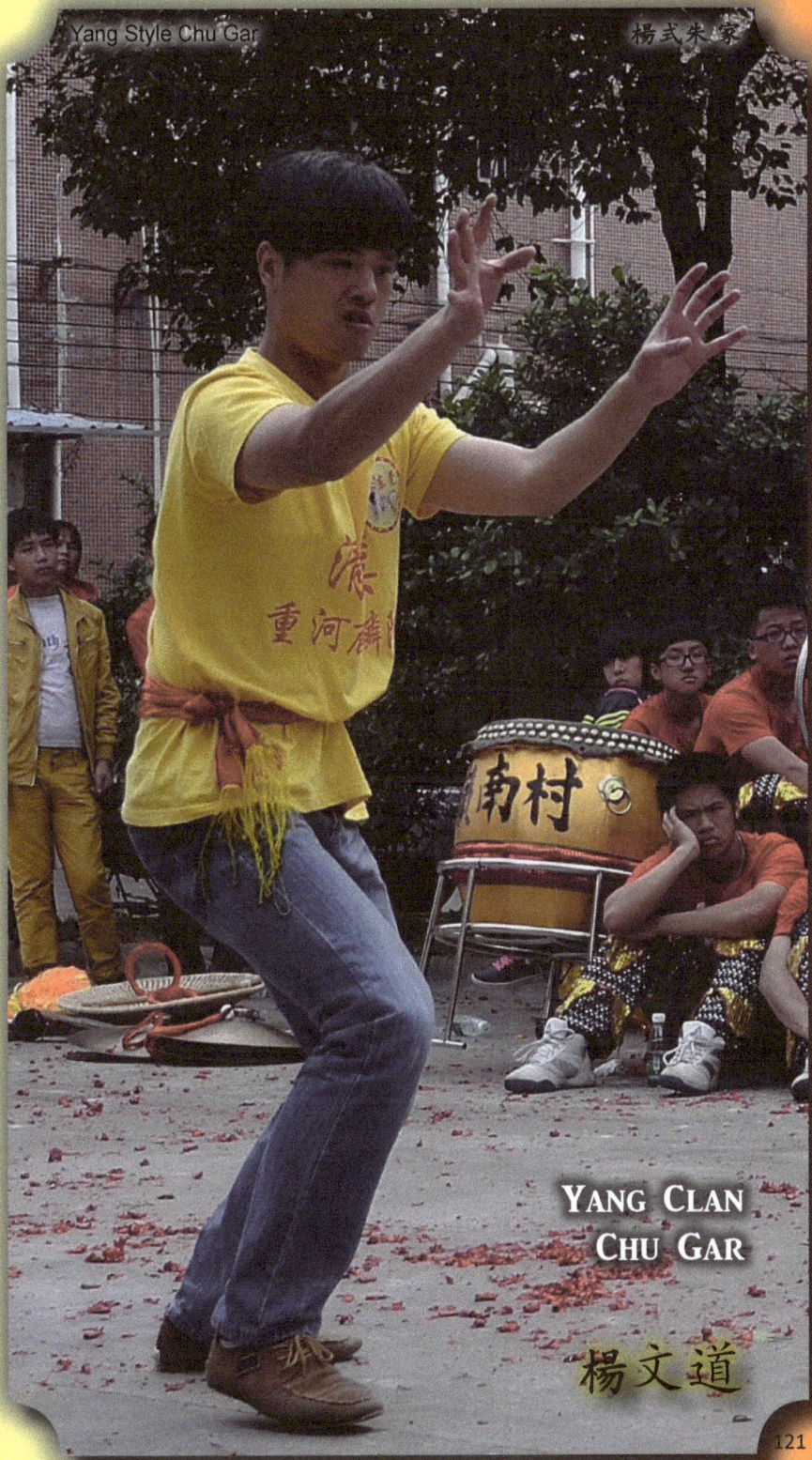

Yang Clan
Chu Gar

楊文道

YANG CLAN CHU GAR

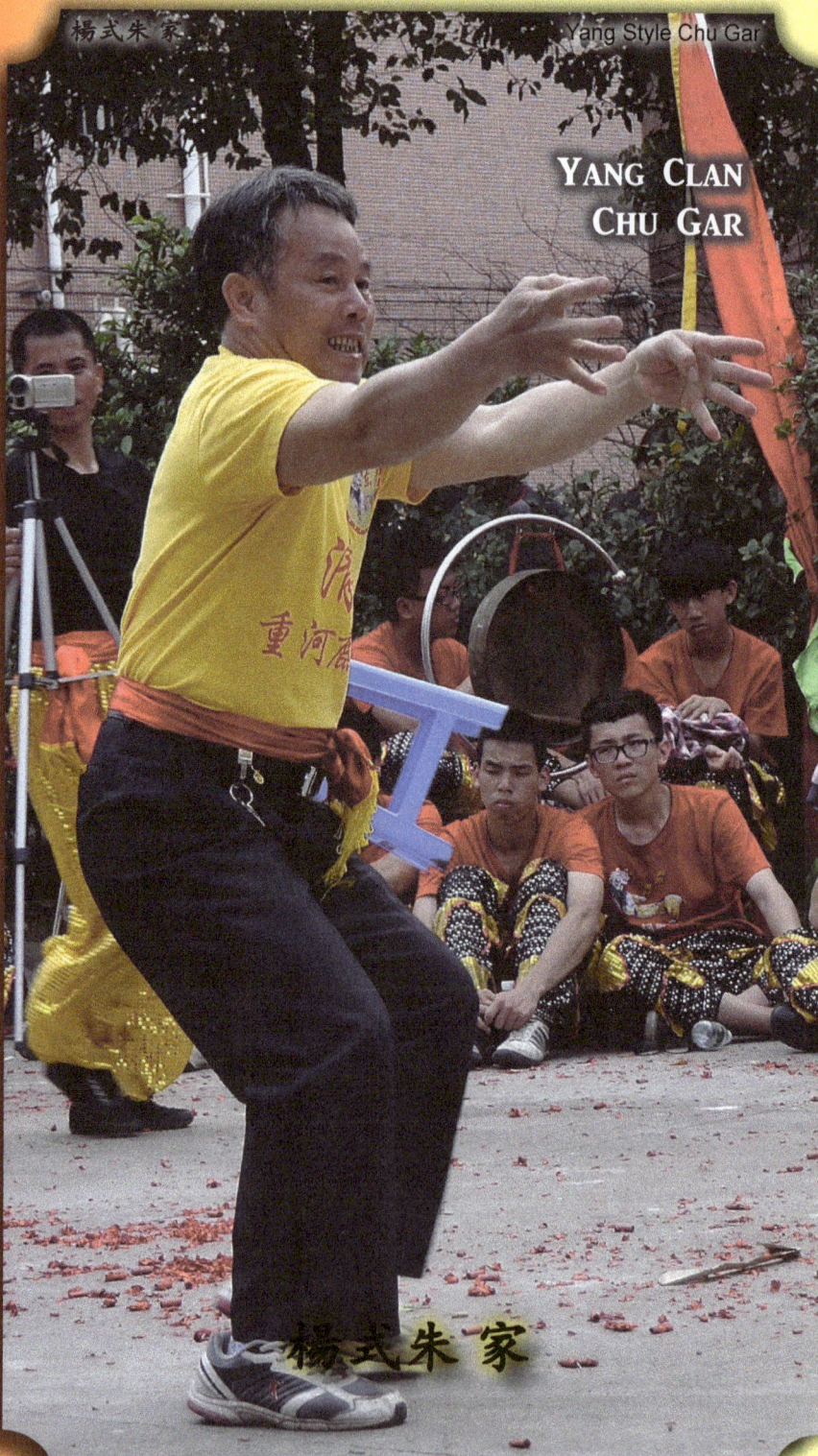

楊式朱家

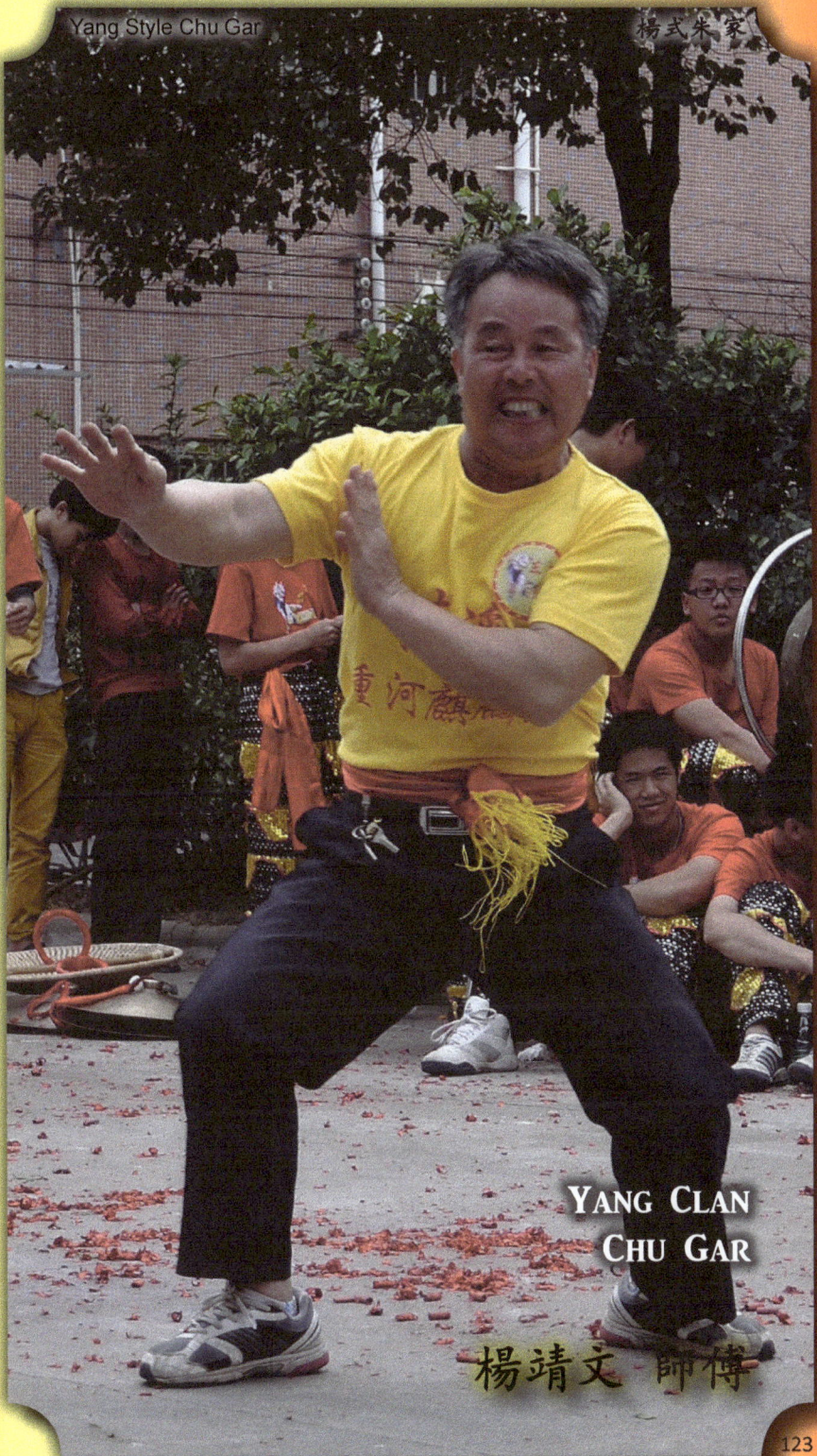

YANG CLAN
CHU GAR

楊靖文 師傅

YANG CLAN
CHU GAR

楊式朱家

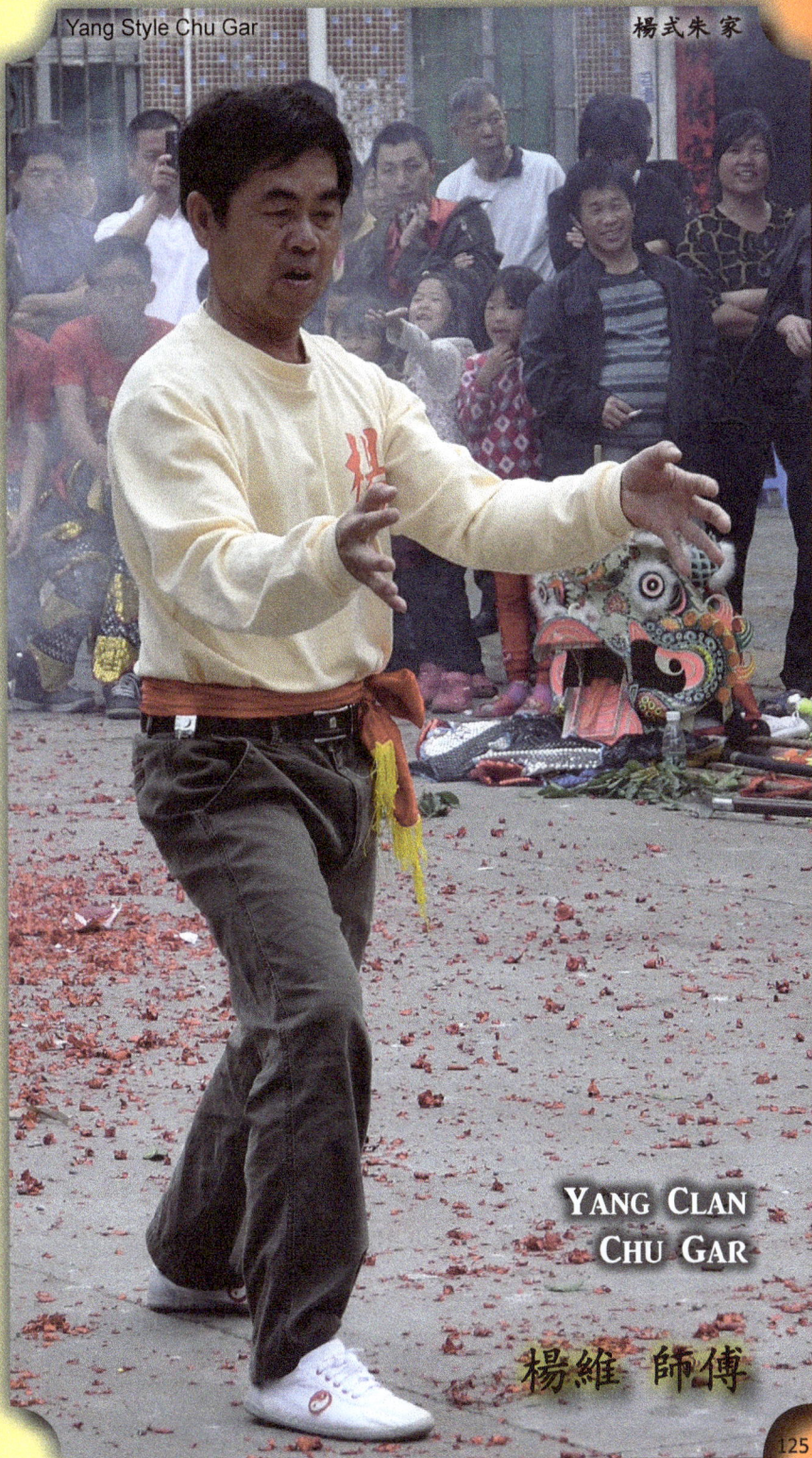

YANG CLAN
CHU GAR

楊維 師傅

YANG CLAN
CHU GAR

楊式朱家

楊式朱家

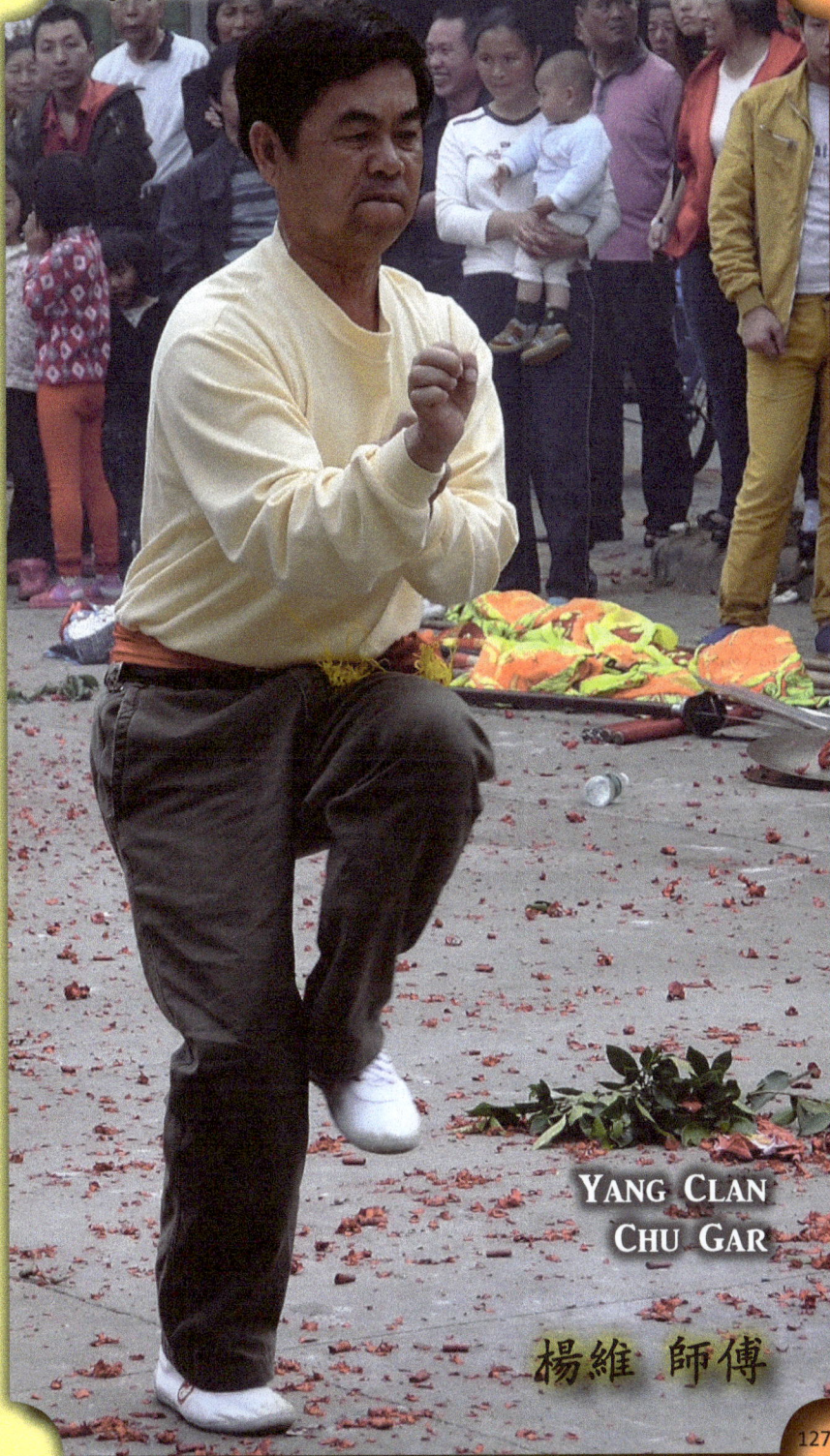

YANG CLAN
CHU GAR

楊維 師傅

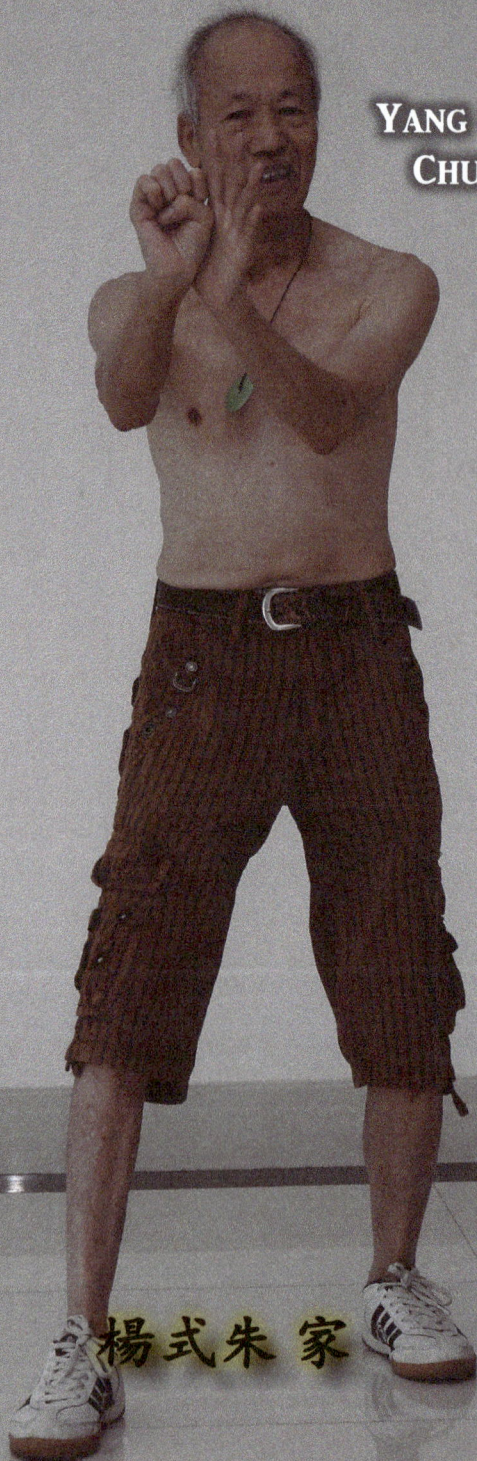

YANG CLAN
CHU GAR

楊式朱家

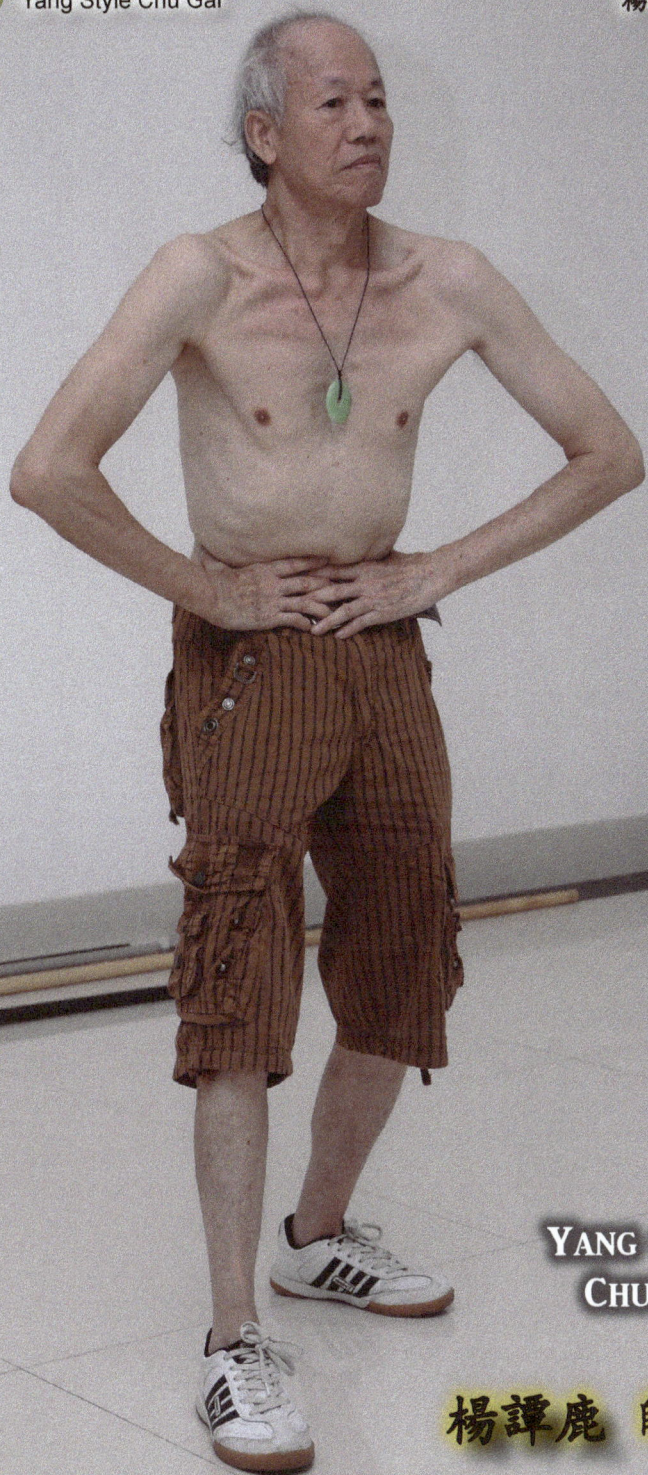

YANG CLAN
CHU GAR

楊譚鹿 師傅

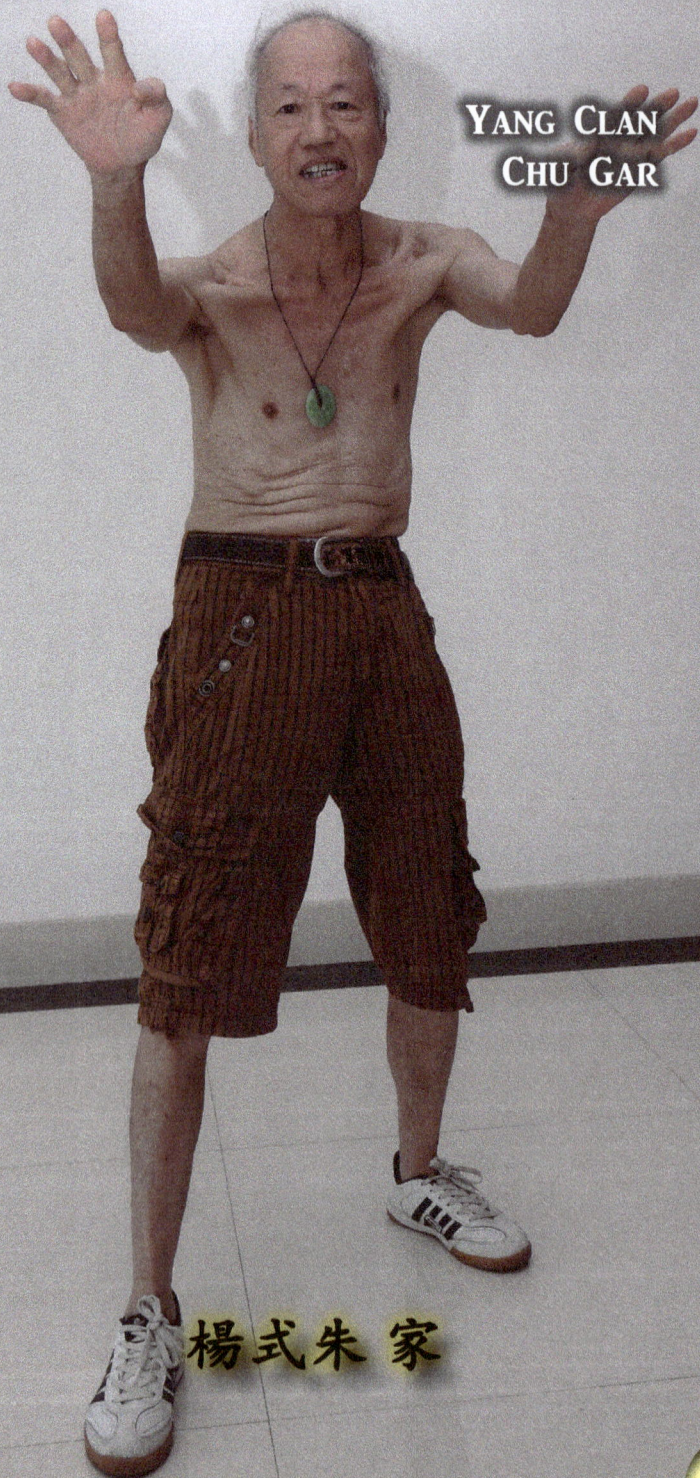

YANG CLAN
CHU GAR

楊式朱家

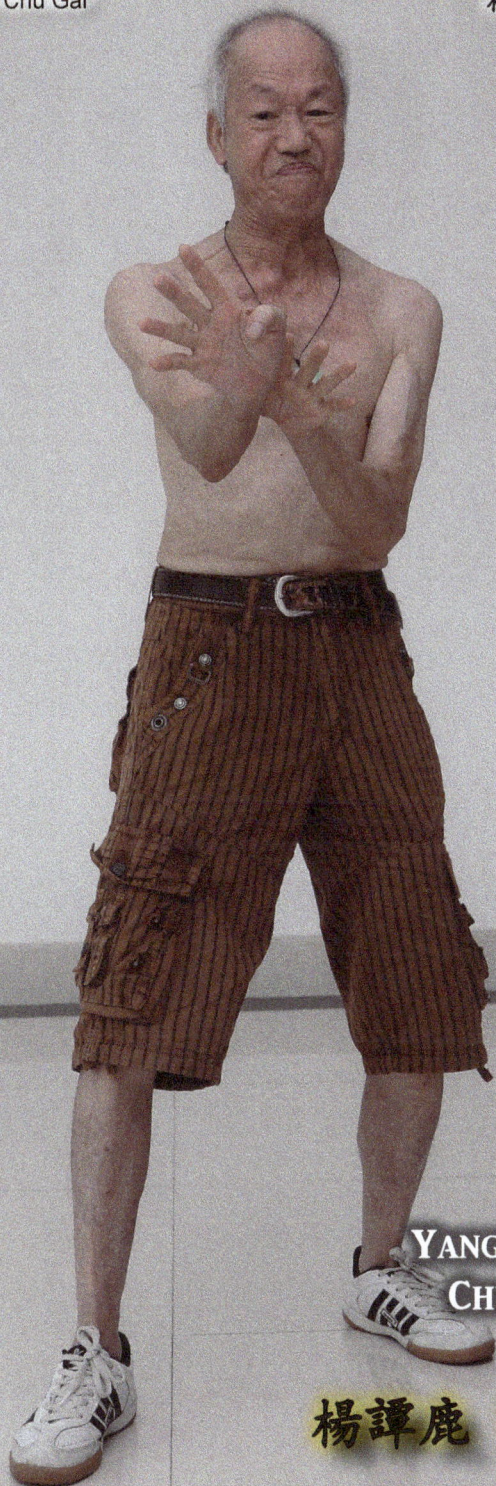

YANG CLAN
CHU GAR

楊譚鹿 師傅

Yang Clan Chu Gar

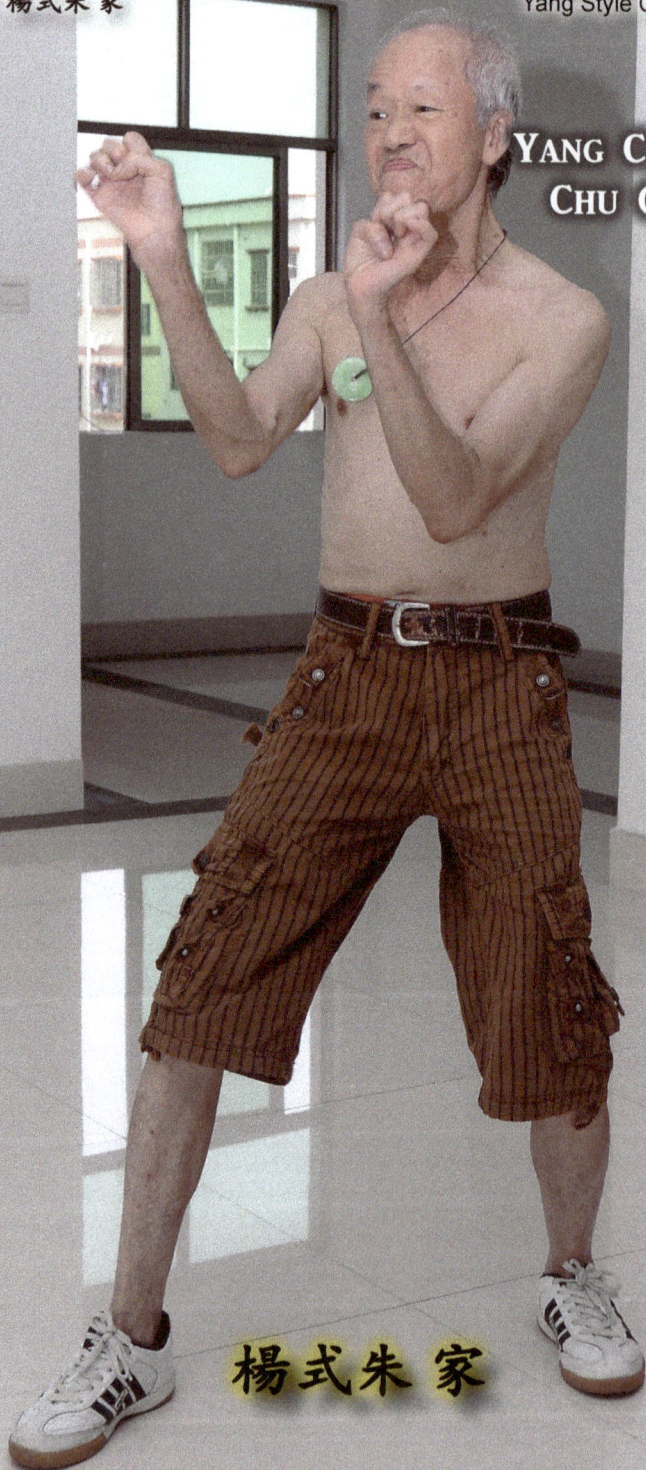

楊式朱家

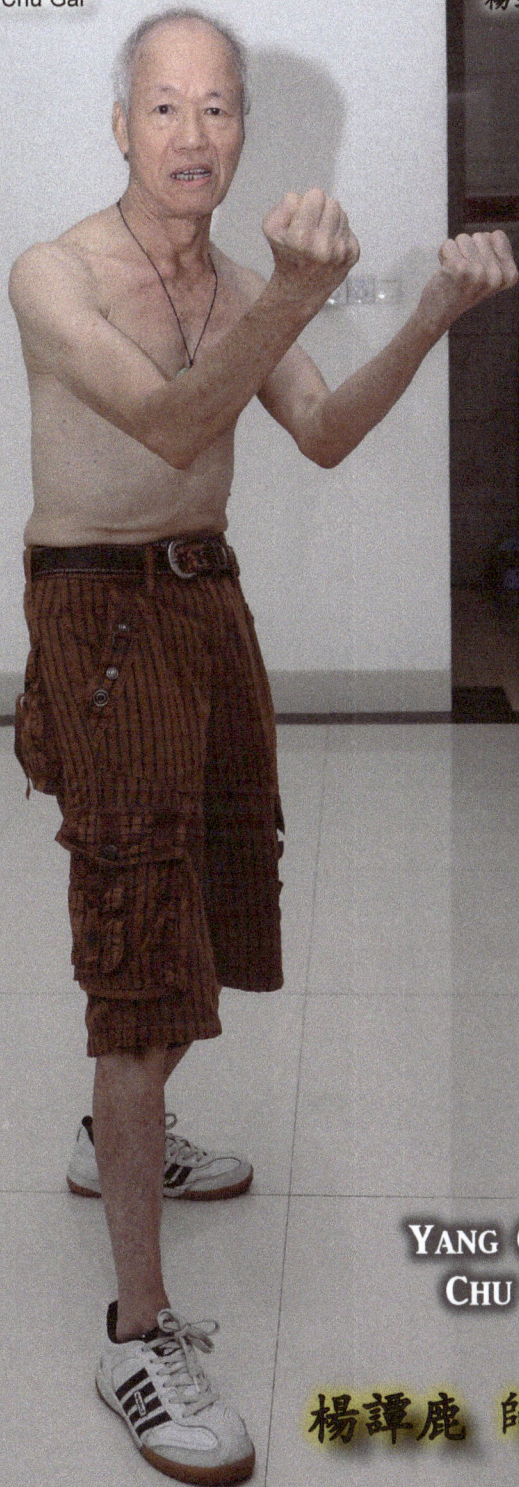

YANG CLAN
CHU GAR

楊譚鹿 師傅

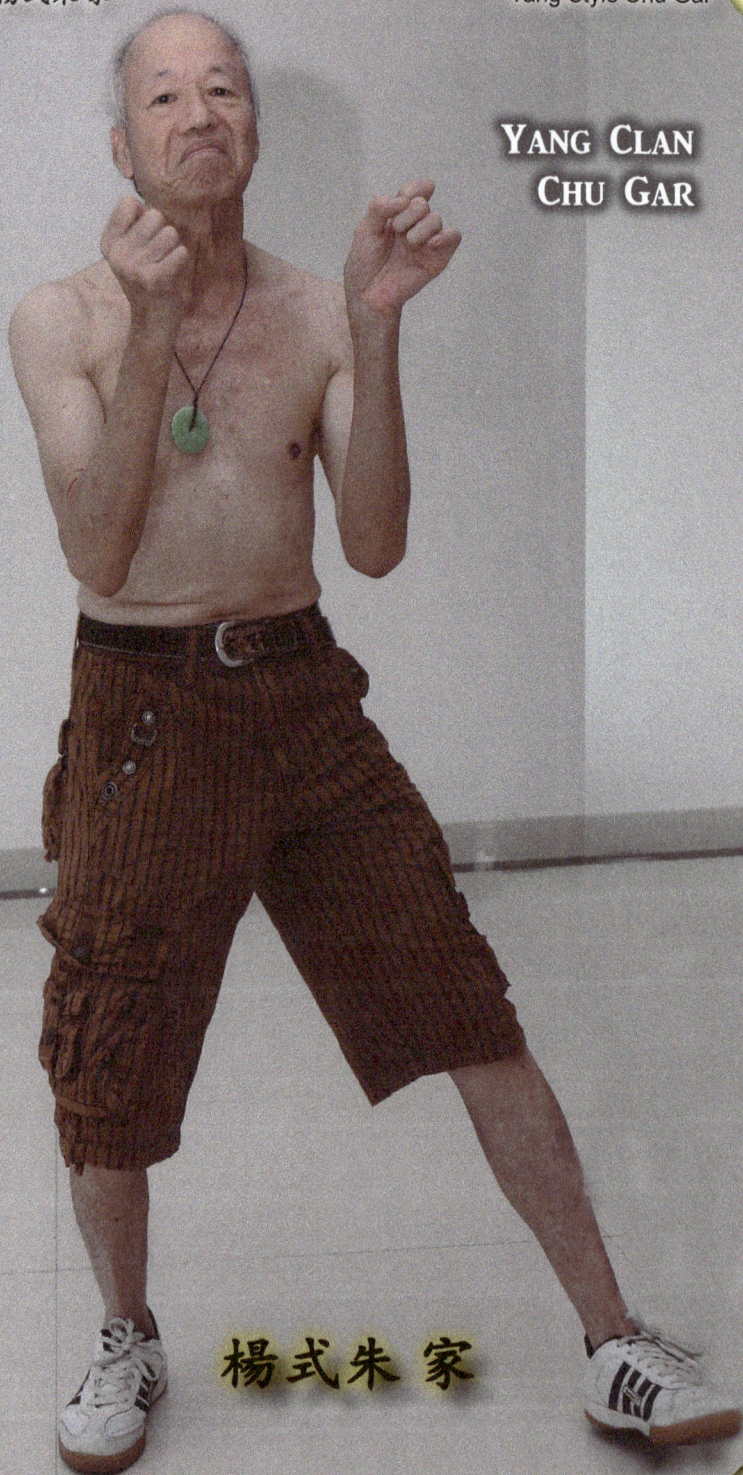

YANG CLAN
CHU GAR

楊式朱家

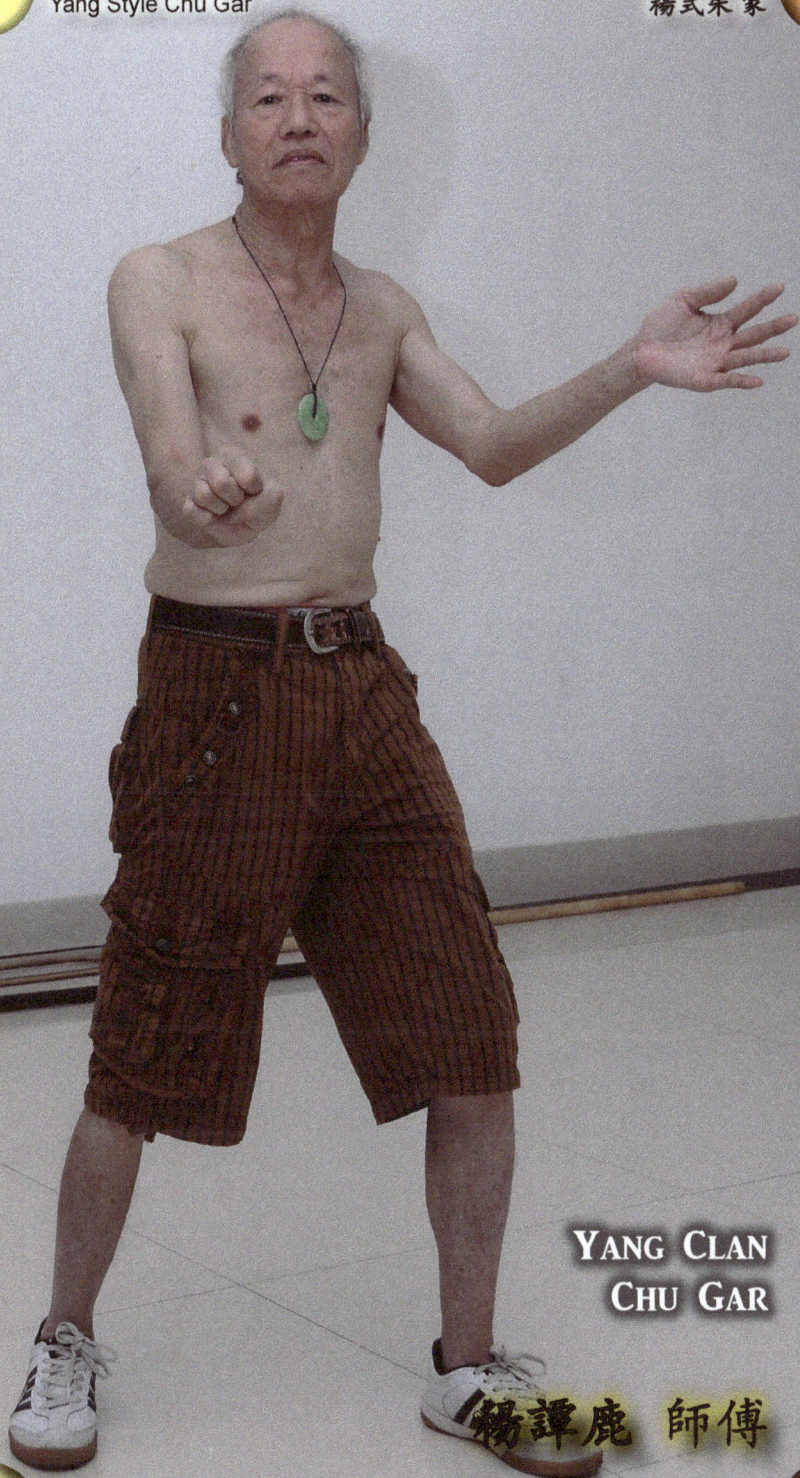

YANG CLAN
CHU GAR

楊譚鹿 師傅

YANG CLAN CHU GAR MANTIS

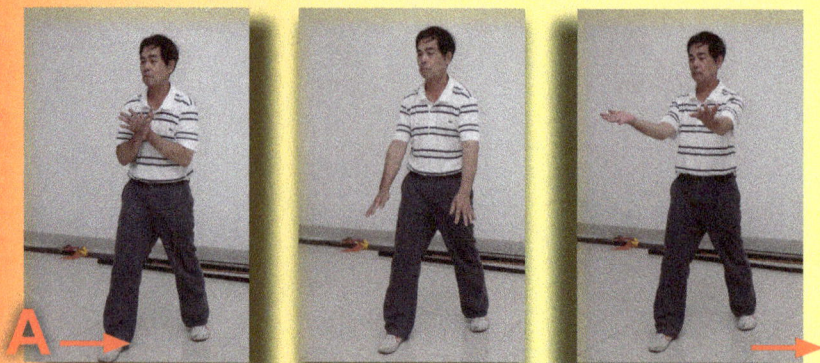

Hand to hand - heart to heart -

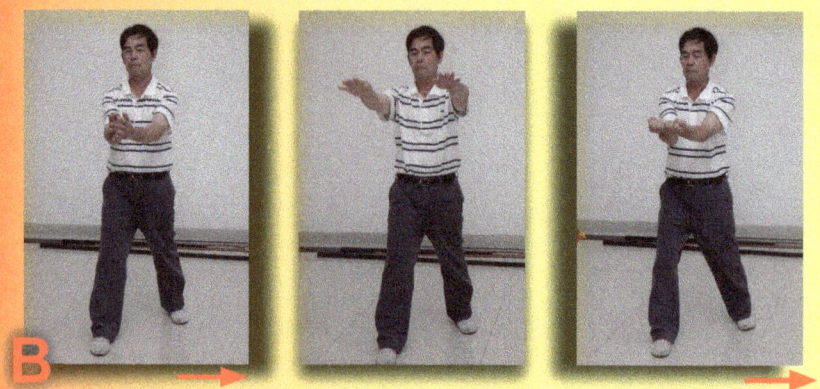

chop shu to clasping hands

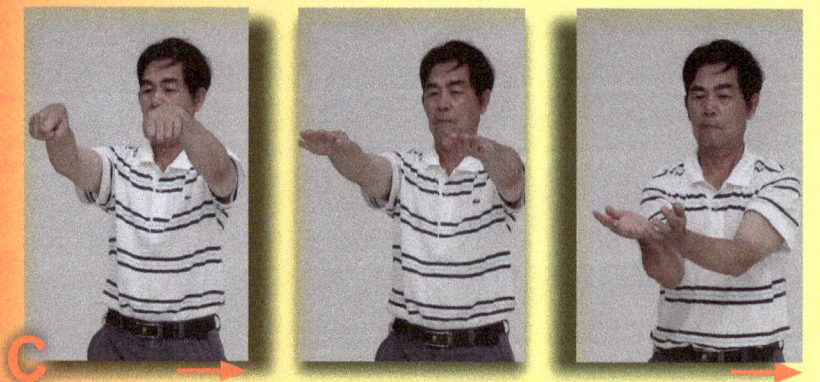

ping- bil - gop mid shot

136

Som Bo Gin Form

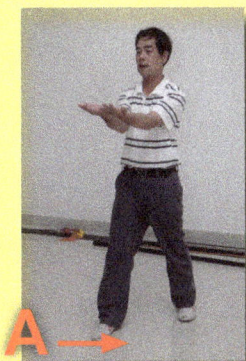
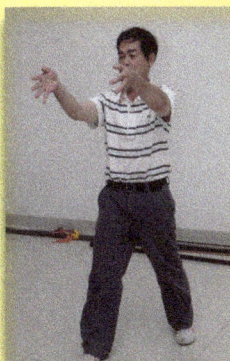
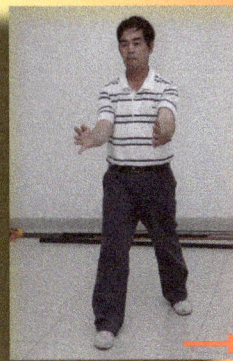

A

hat yi sao beggar's hand to chop shu

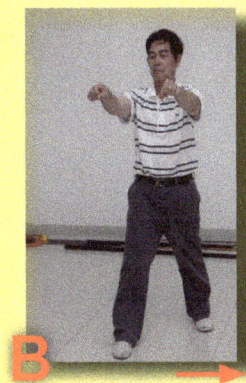
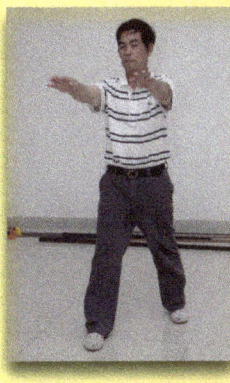
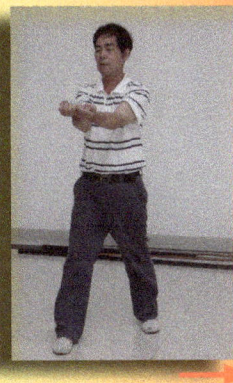

B

ping - bil - gop

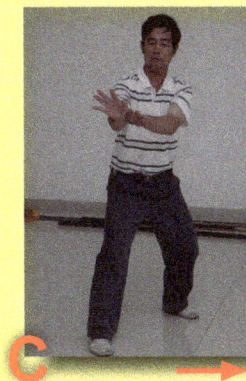
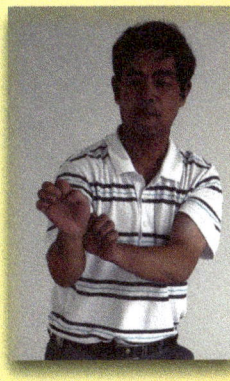
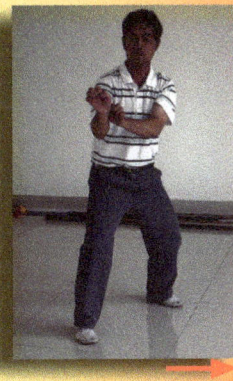

C

lop shu

YANG CLAN CHU GAR MANTIS

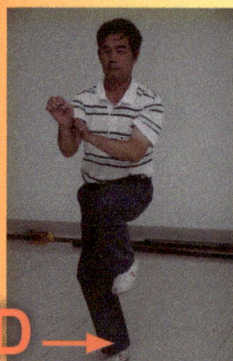

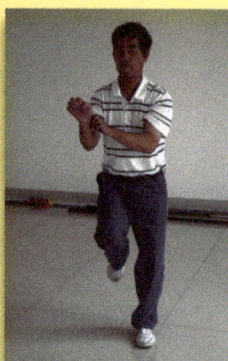

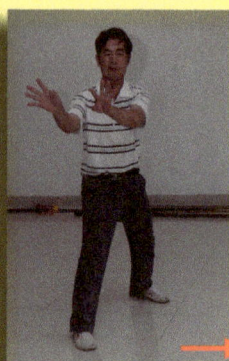

D

lop - double knees - lop sideways

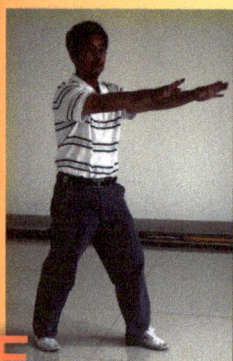

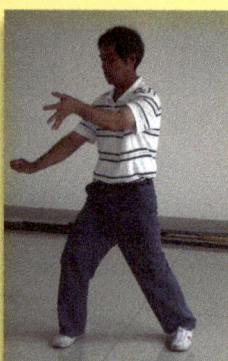

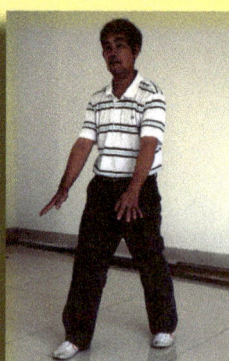

E

lock hands and turn

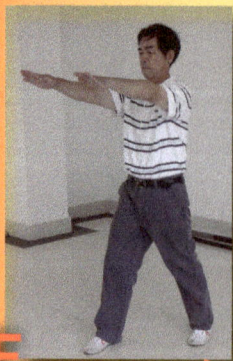

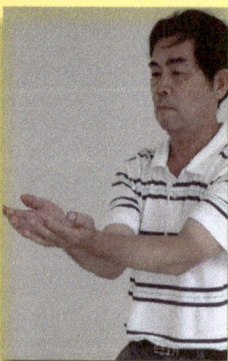

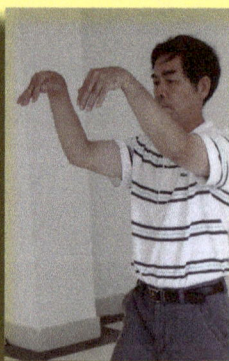

F

bil - gop - ping

楊式朱家

SOM BO GIN FORM

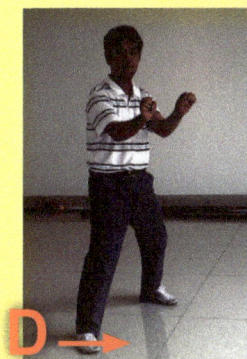

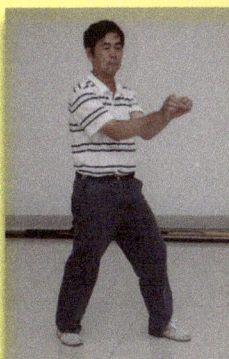

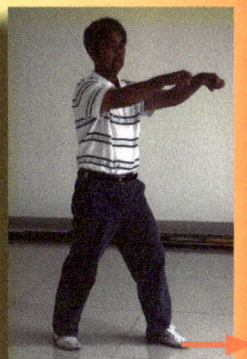

D →

change the angle to 45 off center

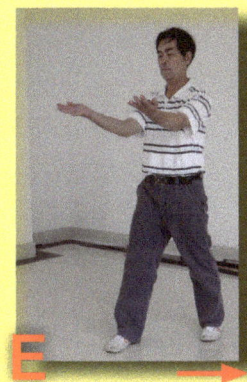

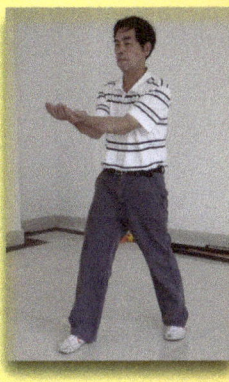

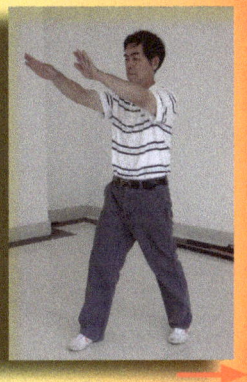

E →

gop and bil jee

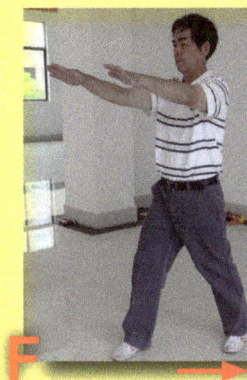

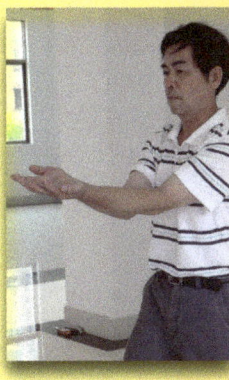

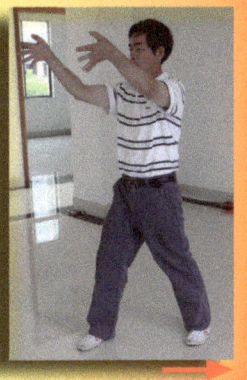

F →

bil - gop - chop

YANG CLAN CHU GAR MANTIS

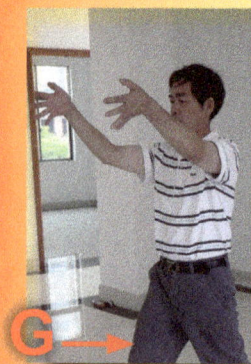

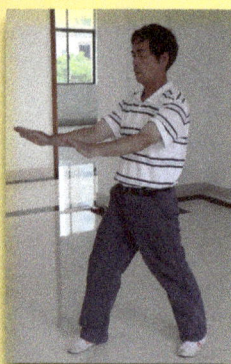

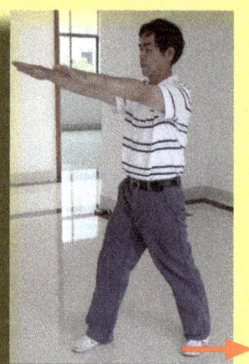

chop - mor - bil

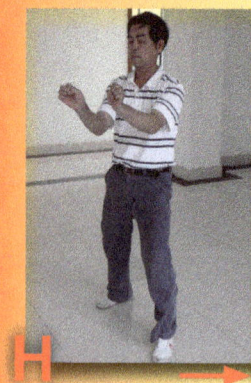

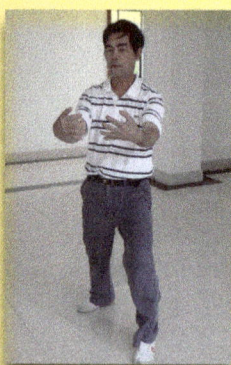

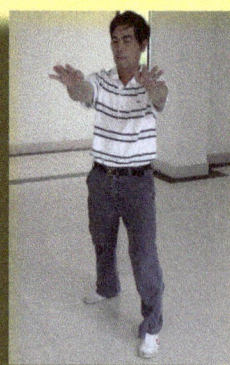

lop - ping zhong - bil

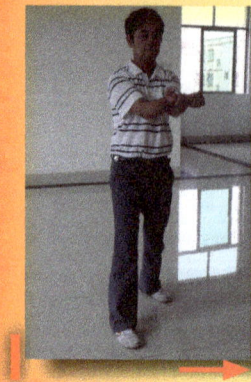

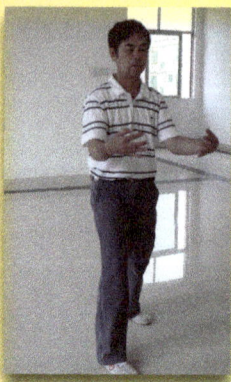

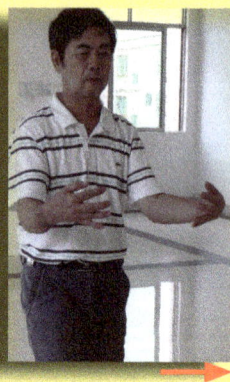

gop - ping zhong

楊式朱家

SOM BO GIN FORM

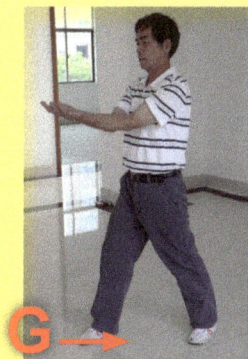

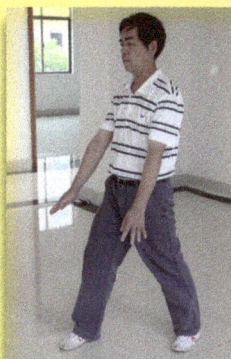

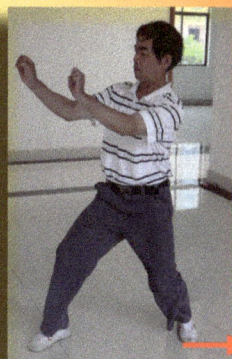

bop - yuan gwak - lop

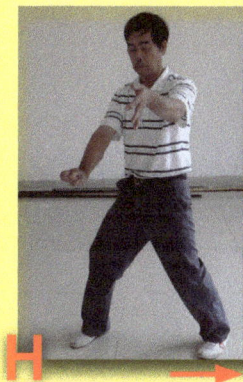

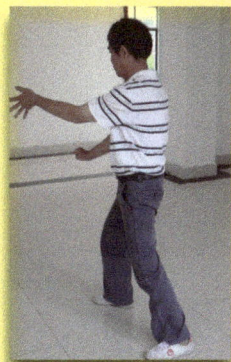

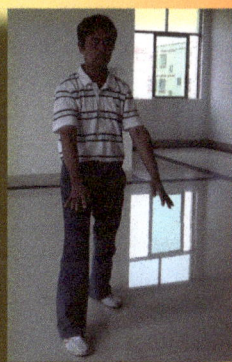

lock hands and turn

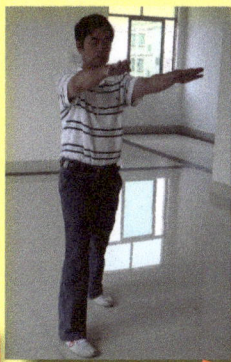

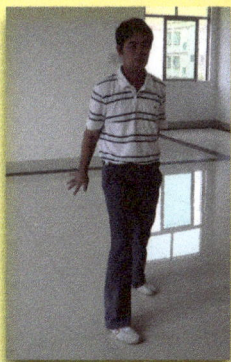

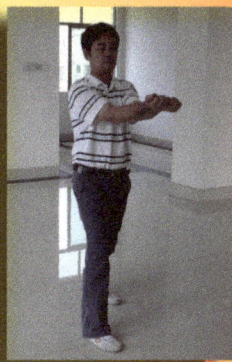

bil - bao hou - not commonly seen in southern mantis

YANG CLAN CHU GAR MANTIS

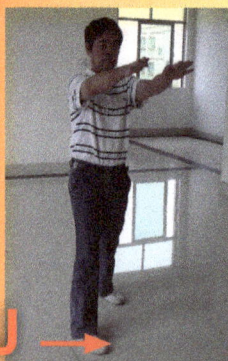

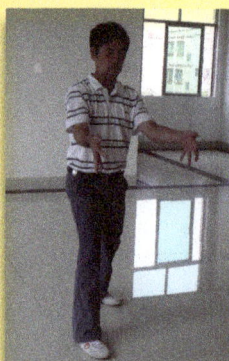

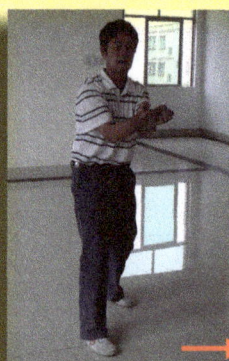

J →

bil - double bridge gwak - gop

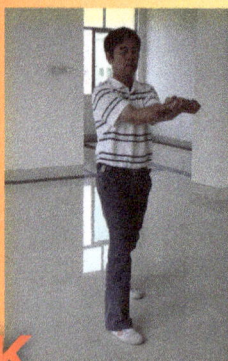

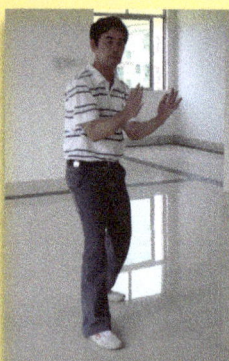

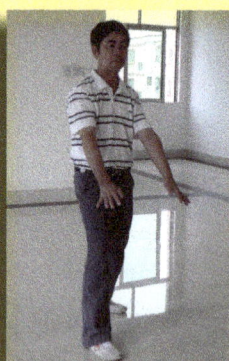

K →

gop - mor - yuan gwak

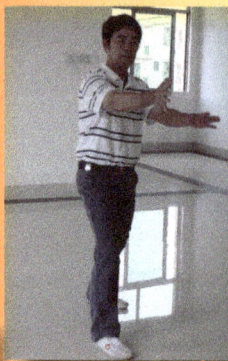

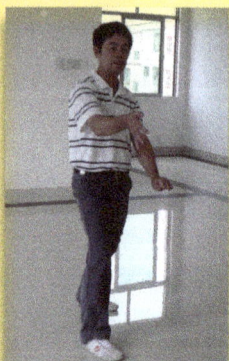

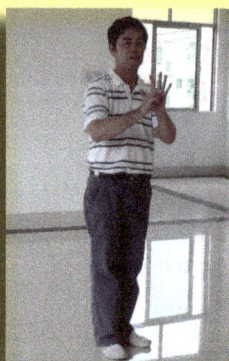

L →

feel - lock - close

SOM BO GIN FORM

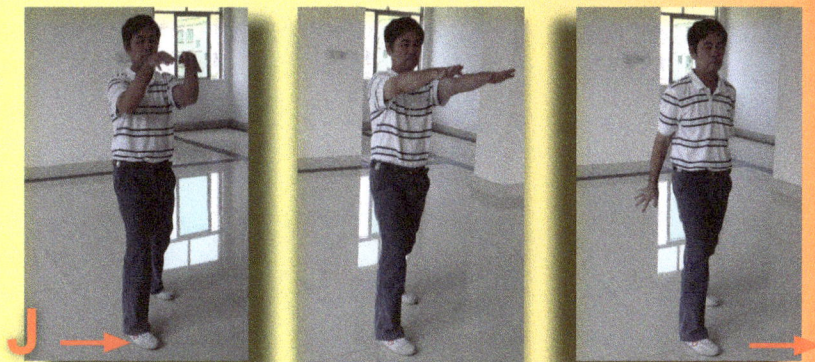

ping - bil - bao hou - not commonly seen in southern mantis

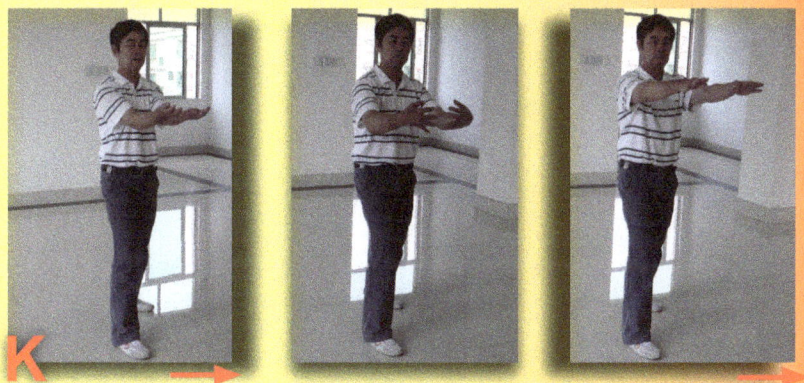

gop - ping zhong - bil

This Yang Style Chu Gar Som Bo Gin form varies significantly from other China, Hong Kong and USA Lam Sang's. It is clear from Yang Wei's up close performance that it is an internal training. He uses abdominal and external musculo-skeletal strength combined overtly and covertly in coordination with his breathing and his facial and emotional expressions.

The form itself can be identified by the hand skills and stepping patterns. It is similar to other Hakka Mantis in that it contains the various hands identified and different in that it contains angular patterns on turn steps not commonly seen and that it contains at the closing sequence double bridge palms to the rear.

This makes an interesting study in origins, strategy and tactics, upcoming. Watch for upcoming media with Yang Wei and the Yang Shou Clan of Chu Gar Mantis.

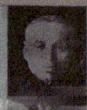

東江朱家螳螂

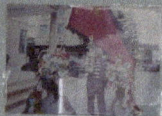 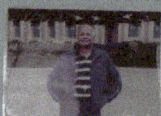 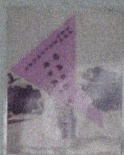

學仁學義學功夫　　　尊親尊師遵教訓

東江朱家螳螂馬步、身形與要訣

馬步身形：丁不丁、八不八、前弓後箭、落地生根、黃蜂腰、竹葉背。

出　拳：拳高三尺、拳由心口發、你不來我不發、你一動我先發、有橋橋上過、無橋自造橋、直來橫接、橫來直破、對方來拳、撥長棄短。

熟　練：攬、拿、抓、提、驚、彈、劾、到時見招化招、心中無招亦有招。

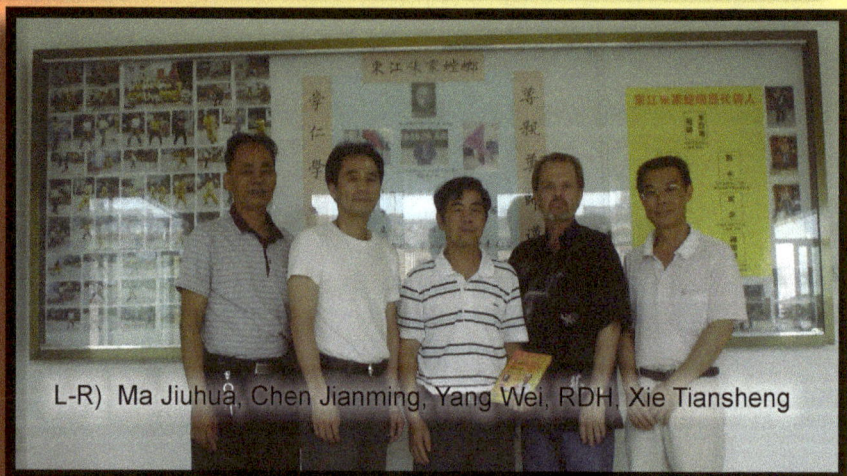

L-R) Ma Jiuhua, Chen Jianming, Yang Wei, RDH, Xie Tiansheng

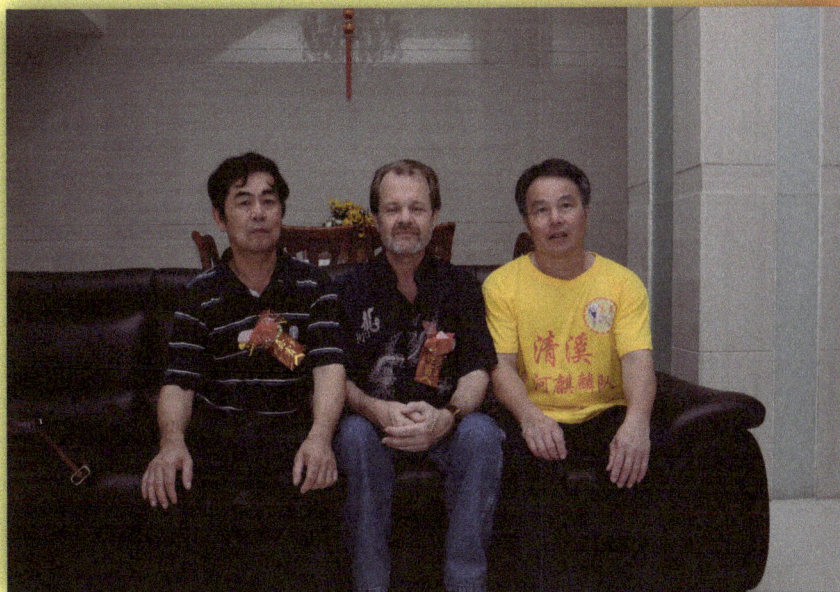

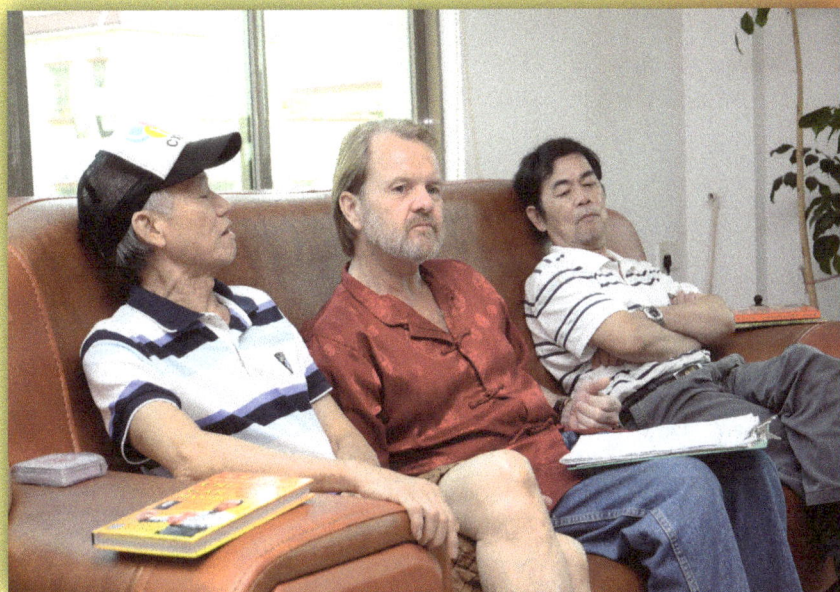

Opposite top: The creed and shrine of Yang Clan Chu Gar
Opposite Bottom: Yang and Huizhou Chu Gar Clans Cooperate
Top: Yang Wei, RDH, Yang Jingwen at Huizhou School Opening
Bottom: Yang HQ - L-R, Yang Tang Lu, RDH, Yang Wei Cooperate

http://southernmantispress.com/spring-summer-2014-news.htm

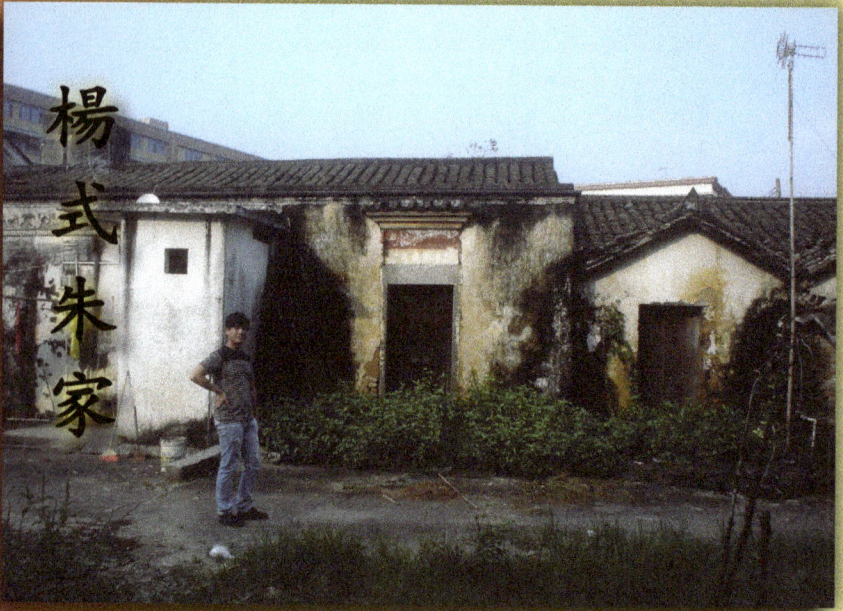

Top: Yang Wen Dao, grandson of the late Yang Shou, first generation disciple of perhaps Wong Fook Go and Lao Sui, surveys Yang Shou's ancestral home from the 1940s.

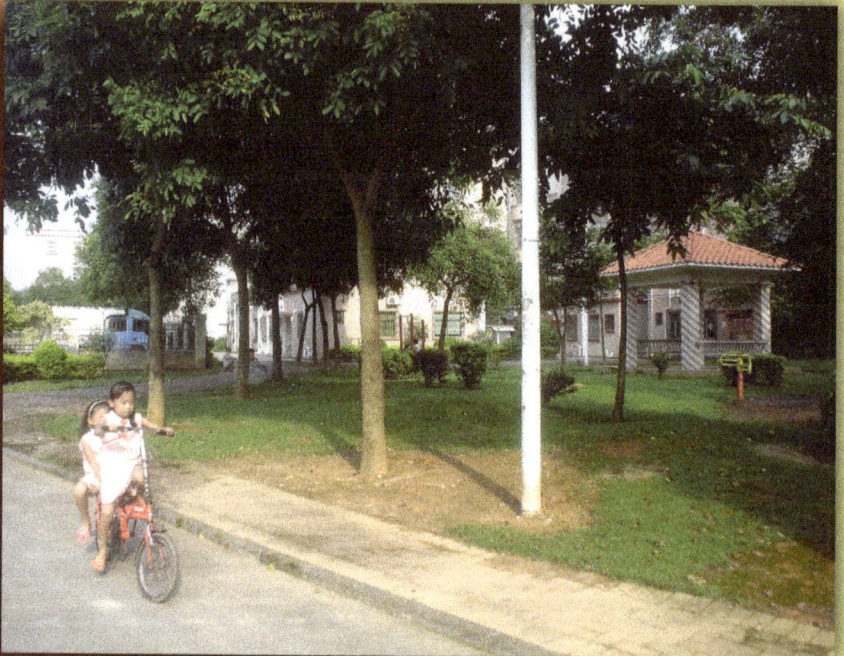

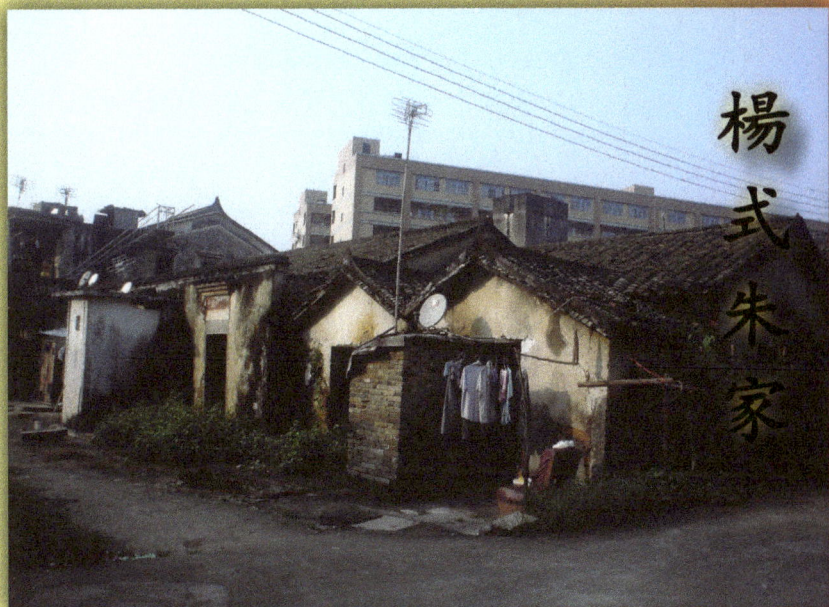

楊式朱家

Opposite Bottom: Many things stand in stark contrast in New China today. Old homes are disappearing as the new quickly replaces the old. Yang Shou's old home is just around the corner from the new Yang Clan Headquarters and in new public parks adjoining the old houses, children play happily.

東江朱家螳螂歷代傳人

Top: The old home of Yang Shou is delapidated and in disrepair, although Yang's transmission of Chu Gar Mantis continues to thrive in his hometown, Qingxi, Dongguan, thanks to those like Yang Wei, Yang Tanglu, and Yang Jingwen.

Bottom: Yang lineage states Yang Shou was a disciple of Wong Fook Go, in Huiyang.

147

Note on Hand Names and Translations
In China, everyone has their own "jia xiang hua", or home town dialect. Hakka is one such dialect and each clan or town may even have their own pronunciation of Hakka language. The names given herein, are the names that are commonly used so that everyone is on the same page and understands which skill or hand is being talked about. It is less important what you call the skills, and more important that everyone understands.

The Chinese romanization herein is the same—it is written phonetically or what is common, so that it can be easily understood. Chinese names herein are not correct pinyin, purposely. All errors in the Chinese text are mine and not to be attributed to the editors.

"Shu, Sao, and Shou" all simply mean "hand" and are often used interchangeably. Remember, once the stance, root and feeling hand is skilled, the whole body is one "hand".

About Southern Mantis on the Internet
The internet and DVDs can be a great aid to learning. How much better are DVDs than secretly peeking through holes in a fence or wall to learn Mantis? In the early days, sneaking a peek through a hole was quite common.

Nothing can replace the spirit and hand of a skillful teacher. But, the new media and resources are still a valuable asset. The internet, however, is also a large source of disinformation. Repeating what someone else said erroneously often becomes accepted as SPM "truth" without verification. There is a great deal of "false" information on the internet about Southern Praying Mantis.

An example is the 'Blanco' article. Circa mid 1990s, Blanco, from Hong Kong, called my office in the USA asking how to contact Southern Mantis teachers in China. I did not provide him any information. Southern Mantis teachers usually frown on unannounced visits from strangers. Later, he "compiled" his article using sources, such as my published works, without permission. Much of his article is erroneous and needs correction. I encourage you to seek the truth for yourself. Do not follow any one blindly. Search and prove all things. The further you go downstream the murkier the water. Drink close to the source.

Errata:
Sifu Ma Jiuhua would like to state clearly that he was misquoted in the Dongjiang Times newspaper. He did not say that Chow Gar did not exist in China and he was misquoted by the reporter. He encourages everyone to come to China and search for themselves. What he said to the reporter was that the legacy of Lao Sui in China is and has always been Chu Gar Mantis from Chu Ya Nan in Wuhua, not Chow Gar. (Refer to my first book, Chu Gar Gao, for more information on the late Sifu Yip Sui and Chow Gar.)

Additional photos indicated ©今日惠州网，天鹅城网

Chu Gar Mantis Today
Many of Lao Sui's relatives train Chu Gar in China today. As stated earlier the Lao and Ma families have been neighbors for more than 100 years and their families have long been related by marriage. The Lao family and Ma families still live side by side in the old village area and both families carry Chu Gar Mantis forward and their ages range from teens to 95 years old. Among the Lao family who train are: Lao Xiang Nan, Lao Yue Gong, Lao Su Shen, Lao Zhen Zhong and Lao Wei Long. Among the Ma family are: Ma Jiuhua, Ma Wei Dong, Ma Yi Liang, Ma Wei Bo, Ma Wei Chao, Ma Wei Liang, Ma Jiu Hui, Ma Wei Ting, Ma Wei Zhen, Ma Wei Cho and others such as Guo Linxiang, Luo Xianming, Zhang Renquan, and Zhen Zihui, etc.

There are three Clans of Chu Gar teaching and all are descended from Ma Mingsen. Sifu Chen Jianming teaches in Huicheng. Sifu Xie Tiansheng in Boluo and Sifu Lin Lunyi in Zhongsan. This is in addition to those who train and teach privately.

Miscellanies

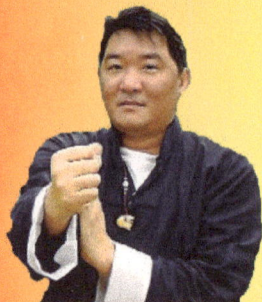

Special thanks to Dr. Simon Han, Taiwan Cardiologist and Weng Chun Boxing teacher, for his time spent editing the Chinese text in this book. You may contact Dr. Han directly by email to discuss Taiwan martial art and for Hakka Mantis training in Taipei, Taiwan - simonclh@gmail.com.

Also, Uncle Cheung Ting and Ms. Huang Yan for their valuable contributions to the Chinese text and this book.

雜記

手法名稱和翻譯

在中國人人有自己的家鄉話或方言。客家話也是一種方言，雖然同屬客家人，但因地理隔閡，客家話的發音及表達用詞常有明顯的出入，

因此我們對每｜手法的名稱和譯名著重於溝通，而非精準而統一的命名，英文音譯名遵循原始方言的發音，但非今日標準漢語拼音，如"shu、 sao, shou"都只是"手"的音譯，經常交互使用。

＊請記住純熟穩固的樁馬和手法將整個身體整合為手。

南方螳螂在互聯網

互聯網和教學光碟對於學習大有助益。但透過教學光碟會比通過柵欄或牆縫偷學更好嗎？在早期偷學是很常見的事。

事實上沒有任何媒體可以取代老師的精神和純熟的手法。但是不可否認的，媒體和網路資源對學習仍然是相當有助益。然而互聯網也是錯誤知識的最大源頭，常見的錯誤就是未經查證而無條件接受別人錯誤的見解，事實上在互聯網上就存在大量的南方螳螂虛假資訊。

大約在 90 年代中期，有人從香港聯繫我，希望我提供中國南方螳螂拳老師的聯絡訊息以便撰寫專文，我沒有提供他任何資訊，因為我知道南方螳螂拳老師通常不喜歡被陌生人打擾，後來

他依循我發表的文章編寫了他自己的文章，可想而知他的文章是錯誤百出，我鼓勵所有對南方螳螂拳有興趣的人自己尋求真理，不要盲從，搜尋並查證所有的資料，應溯溪而上尋找源頭。

勘誤：

馬九華師傅清楚地聲明東江時報的記者對他的訪談有些出入，他鼓勵大家自行來中國查證，他對記者說： 劉水在中國的所傳源自於五華朱亞南的朱家螳螂拳。（參閱我第一本書 "朱家螳螂拳 "後段葉瑞師傅與周家螳螂拳）。

附加照片 © 今日惠州網，天鵝城網

今日朱家螳螂拳在廣東

很多劉水在中國的後人仍學習家傳的朱家螳螂拳，如前文所述的劉水和馬銘森家族比鄰而居且聯姻已經超過百年，他們家族仍居住於劉水故鄉，從十幾歲到九十五歲老人仍然積極練習朱家螳螂拳。他們包括： 劉湘南, 劉瑞光, 劉 Sushen, 劉振忠, 劉威龍; 馬家族人有： 馬九華, 馬偉東, 馬日梁, 馬偉波, 馬偉橋, 馬九良, 馬九輝, 馬偉庭, 馬偉軍, 馬偉珠, 其他為： 郭連相, 羅煜明, 張仁全, 曾志輝, 林潤宇等等。

馬銘森傳人公開教學者則有惠城區陳建明師傅， 博羅的謝添勝師傅和中山的 林潤宇 師傅。 還有其他的一些人。

特別感謝韓志陸博士
(澳大利亞國立昆士蘭大學血管生物學哲學博士)
韓志陸博士為臺北榮民總醫院成人心臟科主治醫師和永春拳教師, 他耗費許多時間翻譯校對本書中文, 您可以直接透過電子郵件 (simonclh@gmail.com) 與他聯絡, 討論武術和客家螳螂拳的訓練。

此外, 還感謝叔叔張庭和女士黃豔為本書的貢獻。

A Final Note

The present is the living sum-total of the whole past. While they still exist, we have the benefit of questioning, hand to hand and face to face, the elders regarding Southern Mantis history and original transmission. However, the elders with first hand knowledge and experience, are less and less with every day passing. Only a handful remain.

This book relates to the basic history of Chu Gar Mantis and Lao Sui's legacy in China. My first Volume, *Chu Gar Gao*, addressed Lao Siu's Chu Gar legacy in Hong Kong.

The three branches of Southern Praying Mantis are from one root. Each has its advantage and is worthy of study. Although, I am first, Kwongsai Jook Lum Temple Mantis, and second, Chu Gar Mantis, both by Ceremony and Transmission, I am not biased or preferential. They are harmonious and may be taught side by side. The only difference is the depth of the transmission one receives.

Train Southern Mantis by DVD or come to Hong Kong and China to study Southern Mantis. Join my class. Email me directly. Welcome!

最后需要注意

目前就是活生生的整个过去的总和。虽然他们仍然存在着，我们有质疑的效益，手手和面对面，关于南部螳螂历史和原始的传输的长老。然而的长老与第一手知识和经验，，越来越少的每一天的传递。只有极少数保持。

这本书涉及到朱家螳螂和刘水遗留在中国的历史。我的第一卷，朱家教，解决刘水朱家遗留在香港。

三个分支的南部螳螂是从一个根。每个有它的优势，是值得研究。虽然我是第一，江西竹林寺螳螂，，第二，朱家螳螂，既由仪式和传输，我没有偏见或优待。他们是和睦的也可以教他们一起。唯一的区别是一个接收的传输的深度。

你想学 DVD 还是来到中国，学南部螳螂，然后你可以直接电子邮件通知我。加入我的课。欢迎您 们！

Roger D. Hagood
Standing Chairman
rdh@chugarmantis.com
www.chugarmantis.com

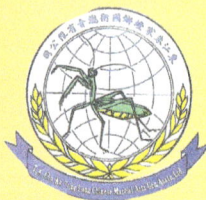

Hong Kong Chu Gar Tonglong Martial Art Association Headquarters

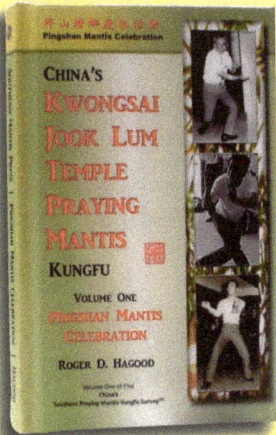

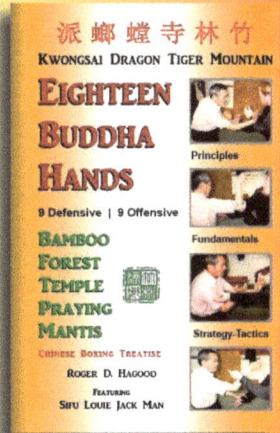

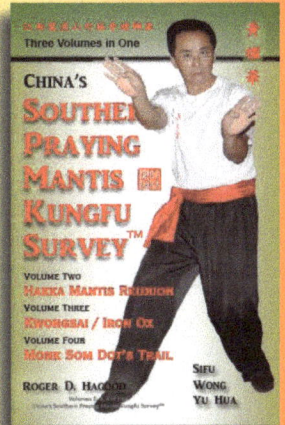

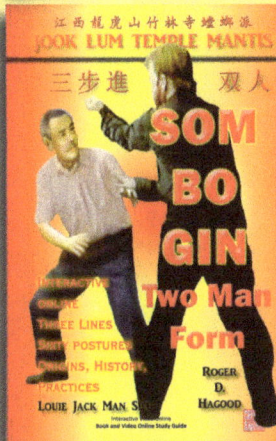

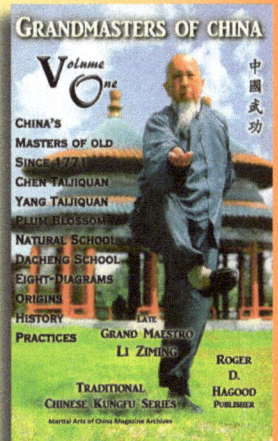

153

Our Family of Hakka Mantis Websites
Visit and Enjoy! Informational, Educational, Instructive

SouthernMantisPress.com
chinamantis.com
bambootemple.com
bambootemple-chicago.com
btcba.com
kwongsaimantis.com
somdotmantis.com
chugarmantis.com
ironoxmantis.com
mantisflix.com
southmantis.com
tientaoqigong.com
oss.tientaoqigong.com
chinamantis.com/youtube
youtube.com/chinamantissurvey

www.southmantis.com/articles/read-rdh-march-mantis-friendship_60.html

**View Online Video Clips of Lao Sui's Village
and Chu Gar Mantis - at the Link Above!**

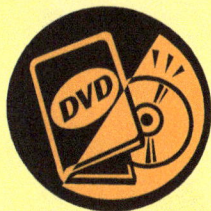

Jook Lum Temple Mantis
Step by Step Instruction
in 18 Volumes

Year One Training

Volume One: Fundamentals; The Most Important
Volume Two: Phoenix Eye Fist Attacking / Stepping
Volume Three: Centerline Defense
Volume Four: One, Three & Nine Step Attack / Defense
Volume Five: Centerline Sticky Hand Training
Volume Six: Same Hand / Opposite Hand Attacks
Volume Seven: Sai Shu, Sik Shu, Jik (Chun) Shu
Volume Eight: Gow Choy; Hammer Fist-Internal Strength
Volume Nine: Footwork in Southern Praying Mantis
Volume 10:   Chi Sao Sticky Hands and Passoffs

Advanced Two Man Forms—Year Two and Three

Available by request. Prerequisite Volumes 1–10.
Volume 11: Loose Hands One
Volume 12: Som Bo Gin
Volume 13: Second Loose Hands
Volume 14: 108 Subset
Volume 15: Um Hon One
Volume 16: Um Hon Two
Volume 17: Mui Fa Plum Flower
Volume 18: Eighteen Buddha Hands
All 8 two man forms must be trained as one continuous set on both A - B sides.

DVD Descriptions and Video Clips

http://www.southernmantispress.com/southern-praying-mantis-instructional-dvds.htm

Summary Year One

http://www.chinamantis.com/first-year-training.htm

聘任證書

香港朱家螳螂鄭運國術體育會

HK CHU KA TONG LONG CHENG WAN MARTIAL ART ASSOCIATION

茲敦聘

ROGER D. HAGOOD

為本會

第廿九屆名譽會長

此聘

香港朱家螳螂鄭運國術體育會

香會會長：馬國蒼
名譽會長：鄭子蘭蒼
名譽會長：朱國威
名譽會長：朱修勤

副主席主席：
副主席主席：夏英國柔術
副主席主席：鄭偉民

國國術副主任：
術副主任：黃國管
副主任：夏國術勤棠起

二〇〇二年 六月中旬 日

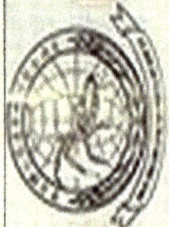

Study Mantis in China with the Author!

Your email correspondence is welcome and do visit and study Hakka Southern Praying Mantis with me in beautiful sunny south China!   I am an Author, Publisher and Producer of eBooks, books, journals, videos and 7 International martial arts newsstand magazines in 15 countries with 48 years in training and teaching martial arts and some 20+ years living in China and Asia!

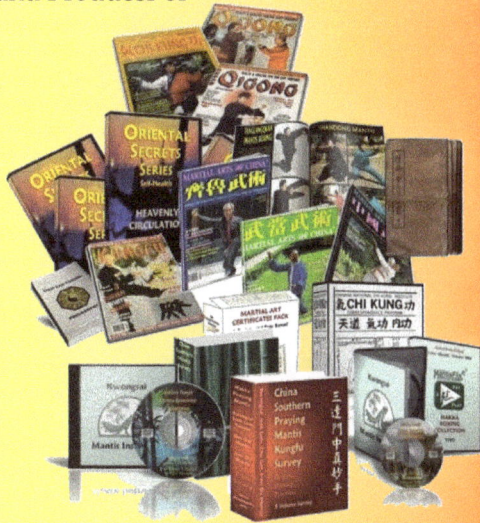

Currently residing in beautiful sunny south China for the last 14 years where I teach Southern Praying Mantis.   Join my class in Guangdong today!

您的電子郵件通信是受歡迎的過來上我的課我教你客家螳螂在美麗陽光南中國！

作者+客家螳螂師傅、 出版商和生產商的電子圖書、 書籍、 期刊、 錄影和 7個 國際武術書報攤雜誌在 15 個國家中有 48 年的培訓和教學武術和一些生活在中國和亞洲的 20+ 年！

目前居住在美麗的陽光南中國那裡我教南部螳螂在過去 14 年。 今天歡迎你們加入我在廣東省的課！

RDH, Pingshan Town, Guangdong, China, Summer, 2015
中國廣東省深圳市坪山鎮2015年夏

More Bio:
http://www.chugarmantis.com/publisher-s-page-2.htm
http://www.chinamantis.com/roger-d.-hagood.htm
Email: rdh@chinamantis.com

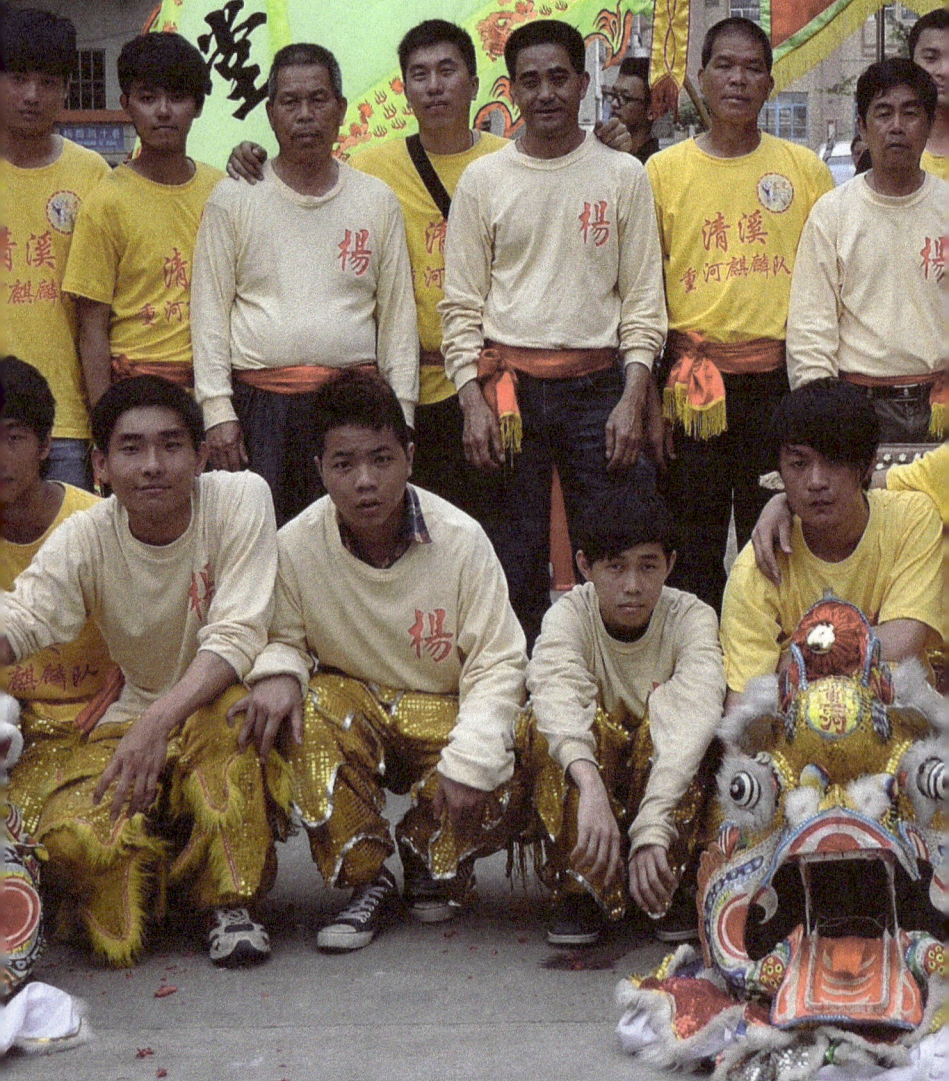

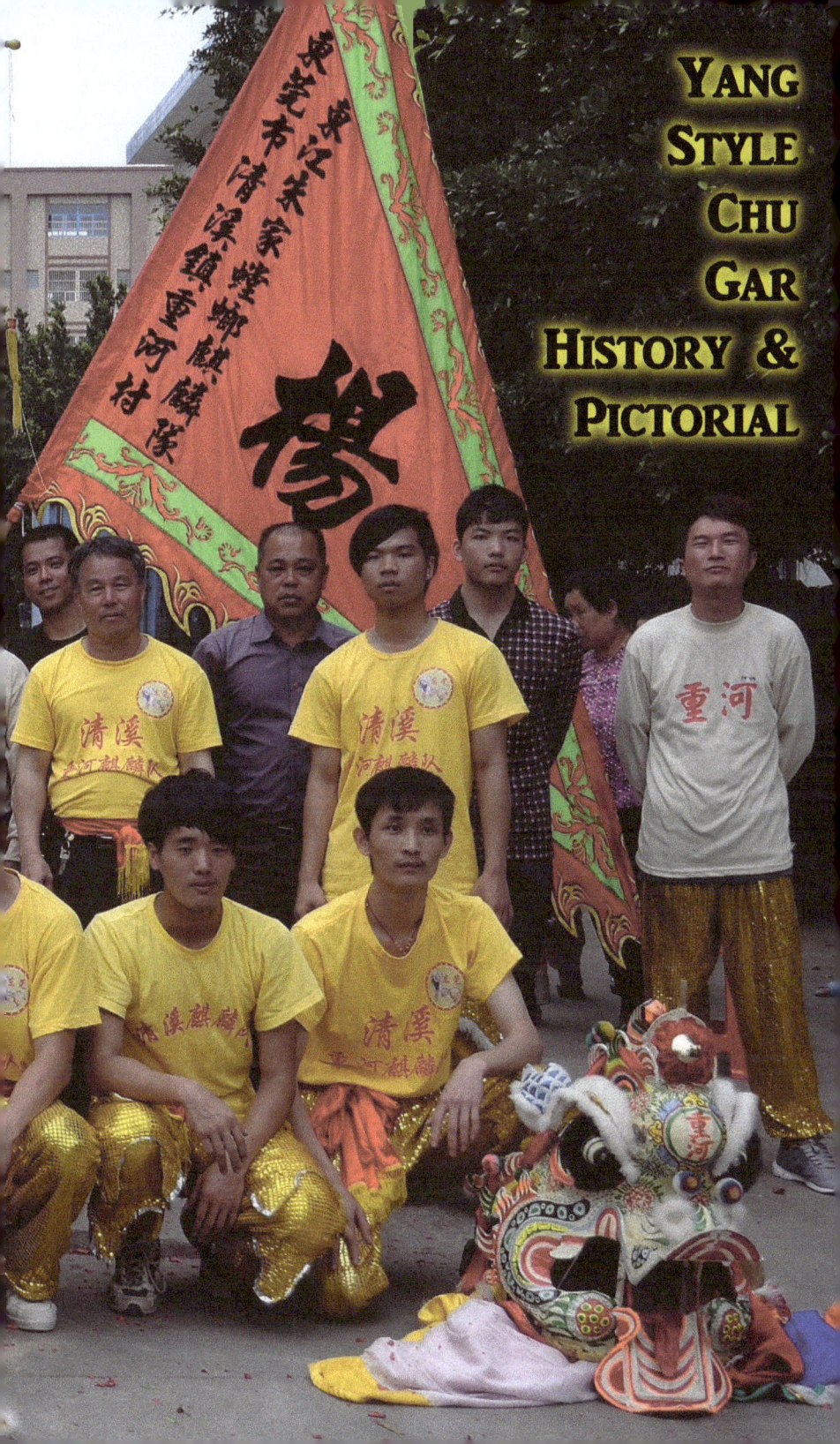

YANG STYLE CHU GAR HISTORY & PICTORIAL